Genereris

PUBLISHING

CHRONIC OBSTRUCTIVE PULMONARY DISEASE AND DEPRESSION

Ivana Jelić
Goran Mihajlovic

Title: CHRONIC OBSTRUCTIVE PULMONARY DISEASE AND DEPRESSION

ISBN: 979-8-89966-044-3

Author: Ivana Jelić, Goran Mihajlovic

Cover image: www.pixabay.com

Publisher: Generis Publishing
Online orders: www.generis-publishing.com
Contact email: info@generis-publishing.com

CONTENTS

It is estimated that the incidence of chronic obstructive pulmonary disease has doubled or even tripled since the 1960s. In fact, today it is estimated that around 300 million people worldwide suffer from it. What is most concerning is the fact that this number is constantly increasing. Patients with chronic obstructive pulmonary disease (COPD) have a wide range of comorbidities, and depression is the least studied. Mood disorders have a high comorbidity potential, more so than other mental or physical illnesses. For these reasons, increasing attention is being paid to screening programs in primary health care, although a single "screening" diagnostic instrument for the assessment of depression in COPD has not yet been developed. Instruments such as the Beck Depression Inventory and the Hamilton Depression Rating Scale are the most used [Lim SU et al., 2019; Park K et al., 2020; Kondo K et al., 2020; Obeid S et al., 2023]. The 2017 WHO recommendations emphasize the importance of screening all patients over the age of 18 in primary care for depression. This includes all chronically ill patients [WHO, 2017].

There are various obstacles to detecting depression in COPD patients, both by patients themselves and by doctors. The most common barrier that patients have is the "stigma" that exists about mental illnesses, refusal to reveal symptoms and lack of knowledge about the diseases. Doctors are increasingly emphasizing the importance of educational counseling centers, believing that through education they will bring patients closer to the importance of preventive examinations and reduce the level of mental disorders [WHO, 2017; WHO, 2021].

There are no precise data on the prevalence of depression in COPD, because there is no single instrument for assessing depression, and because of different degrees of consideration of chronic obstructive pulmonary disease in different studies. Less than 50% of patients with depression are recognized, which indicates the need to identify patients with chronic obstructive pulmonary disease with comorbidity of depression in the early phase of the disease. A simple and quick way to detect symptoms of depression is to use an adequate questionnaire [Urtasun M et al., 2019; Story DA et al., 2019; Morin A, 2021; APA, 2023; Ayalon L et al., 2010; Manea L et al., 2012], which will be discussed later in this book.

PART ONE
Chronic Obstructive Pulmonary Disease

1. Chronic Obstructive Pulmonary Disease – Definition

COPD is a well-defined disease, thanks to the availability of medical methods and respiratory centers where studies are performed. However, it remains an unrecognized, underdiagnosed and undertreated disease globally [GOLD, 2021].

Data from the European Association for Chronic Lung Diseases, especially in developing countries, indicate that COPD is a preventable and treatable disease. The Global Strategy for the Diagnosis, Treatment and Prevention of COPD defines chronic inflammatory lung disease as a complex, non-reversible airflow limitation that is invasive and associated with a chronic inflammatory response of the lungs to noxious particles and gases [GOLD, 2021].

At the heart of airflow limitation is inflammation that occurs in the small airways and lung parenchyma. The destruction of the parenchyma, which occurs as part of the inflammatory response, leads to a decrease in lung elasticity with the destruction of the lung parenchyma and the development of emphysema [Hogea SP et al., 2020].

The main symptoms of COPD are cough, expectoration, dyspnea, and symptoms of increased fatigue. Dyspnea is usually persistent and progressive. Initially, dyspnea is associated with heavy physical work, and later it manifests itself with less and less physical effort, while ultimately it becomes difficult to perform even the most basic daily activities [AIHW, 2020].

It is assumed that in patients with COPD, dyspnea, inactivity, and loss of physical fitness led to even greater inactivity, social isolation, fear and the onset of depression. Such patients often feel useless, show a strong dependence on others in terms of caring for their own health and overall life, they lose interest in future events, and the like.

However, these symptoms may not develop until significant lung damage occurs, especially if the patient continues to be exposed to risk factors [Cohen BH et al., 1997; Brashier BB et al., 2012; GOLD, 2023].

The clinical diagnosis of COPD is based on symptoms such as dyspnea, chronic cough, sputum production, exposure to risk factors, and spirometry.

Spirometry-based severity assessment:

COPD is classified into four stages according to the GOLD criteria [GOLD, 2023], based on the forced expiratory volume in one second – FEV1 (Table 2).

Dyspnea assessment:

When assessing dyspnea, GOLD recommends using the Modified British Medical Research Council (mMRC) dyspnea scale (Table 3) [GOLD, 2023].

1.1. Epidemiological Trend in Chronic Obstructive Pulmonary Disease

In observing the epidemiological trend of COPD, prevalence, morbidity and mortality are considered.

Despite numerous studies, available data on the prevalence of COPD are very different. Globally, the prevalence is 11.7% [AIHW, 2020]. In terms of prevalence in different groups of countries, an increase in prevalence is observed in middle-income countries, and it reaches very high values in developed countries.

Consumption of nicotine in larger quantities is one of the main factors for the development of obstructive pulmonary disease [Hogea SP et al., 2020]. Meta-analytic studies have proven that excessive consumption of nicotine combined with genetic predisposition is a major factor in the development of lung damage. In the United States of America (USA), systemic diseases caused by excessive consumption of nicotine are the most common cause of morbidity and mortality. In the 18-46 age group, two-thirds of the respondents continuously consume nicotine and hard alcoholic beverages, of which 60-90% of patients report anamnestic data on continuous consumption of nicotine for a long period of time [Hogea SP et al., 2020; AIHW, 2020; Lazic Z et al., 2021]. Smoking 30-40 cigarettes per day for six to twelve years often leads to lung obstruction with destruction of the lung parenchyma [WHO, 2025]. The age of the patient, the severity of the clinical picture, the results of laboratory tests and the results of diagnostic procedures are most often considered when assessing the severity of COPD [GOLD, 2018; Zareifopoulos N et al., 2019].

The authors conducted a study of 8387 patients with chronic diseases. They showed that chronic obstructive pulmonary disease is most often associated with depression. Depression occurs in 26.6% of patients with COPD, and most patients are older than 55. The study lasted 10 years. Follow-up was performed every two years. The occurrence of depressive symptoms after the diagnosis of one of seven chronic diseases, including COPD, was considered. It was noted that after two years from the diagnosis of COPD, the hazard ratio for the development of depression was 2.21, for cancer 3.55, and for heart disease 1.45 [Polsky D et al., 2005].

Depression is most often associated with younger age, female gender, smoking, cough, and cardiovascular disease. In stable COPD, the prevalence of depression ranges from 10-42% [Umareta NR, 2023]. Patients with severe COPD, on long-term home oxygen therapy (62%) are particularly at risk [Oswald-Mammosser M et al., 1995; Wijesinghe M et al., 2011; Hardinge M et al., 2015].

In patients with exacerbations, the prevalence of depression is higher and ranges from 19.4% to 50% [Tselebis A et al., 2010; Annavarapu M et al., 2015]. Some studies estimate the prevalence to be 6-59%. Post-hoc testing was used to analyze 64 studies that included patients with severe COPD, where the prevalence of depression varied between 37-71% and was even higher compared to the prevalence of depression in patients with asthma, cancer, heart disease, and kidney disease [Bozkurt N et al., 2022; Long J et al., 2020; Mold E et al., 2010].

Morbidity data indicate different frequencies of COPD worldwide, and it is estimated that around 300 million people suffer from it. What is most worrying is the fact that this number is constantly increasing. Namely, in many countries this number has doubled or even tripled in recent years. Patients have a reduced quality of life, and factors that significantly affect the ruined health condition are the severity of the disease, the use of long-term therapy, comorbidities, frequent exacerbations and frequent hospitalizations [GOLD, 2018].

As indicated in the available scientific literature, COPD is a chronic disease in which prevalence and mortality are constantly increasing. Therefore, this disease is among the top ten leading causes of death in the world. More precisely, COPD is the third leading cause of death in the world and in countries with upper middle income and fourth in countries with lower middle income. According to WHO, COPD is expected to be the third leading cause of death by 2030 [WHO, 2021].

1.2. Risk Factors for Chronic Obstructive Pulmonary Disease

The risk factors that lead to the destruction of the lung parenchyma and impaired airflow through the lungs are numerous. COPD most often occurs because of the interaction of genetic and environmental factors. The most significant risk factors for COPD are active and passive smoking, air pollution, infections, genetic risk, diet, and poor socioeconomic status. Risk factors are divided into factors that contribute to the development of the disease and factors that are triggers for the onset of COPD symptoms (Table 1). Often, these factors act together to develop chronic inflammation in the lung parenchyma [GOLD, 2013; Antuni JD et al., 2016].

Table 1. Factors leading to the development and expression of COPD

A. Risk factors
Smoking cigarettes (active and passive) Exposure to biomass smoke Occupational exposure Air pollution
B. Predisposing factors
Genetics Female gender Low socioeconomic status
C. Childhood adversity
Intrauterine growth restriction Low birth weight Severe childhood respiratory infections
D. Lung conditions
Airway hyperresponsiveness Asthma Chronic mucus hypersecretion Recurrent bronchopulmonary infections Emphysema detected on high-resolution computed tomography

Source: Adapted from [Antuni JD et al., 2016]
https://www.ncbi.nlm.nih.gov/pmc/articles/PMC5556761/

Meta-analytic studies have shown that excessive nicotine consumption, combined with genetic predisposition, is a major factor in the development of lung damage [Zhou X et al., 2012; Dome P et al., 2010]. Nicotine is one of the most harmful components of tobacco smoke [U.S. Department of Health and Human Services, 2014; Marsh S et al., 2006; Hikichi M et al., 2019; Lamprecht B et al., 2011; Di Rosanna P et al., 2012]. When tobacco smoke is inhaled, nicotine is rapidly absorbed through the pulmonary alveoli and is mainly metabolized in the liver (80-90%), and to a lesser extent in the kidneys and lungs [Benowitz NL et al., 1998; Yoshida T et al., 2007; Jain D et al., 2021]. Active smoking produces carbon monoxide, which is retained in the lungs and leads to destruction of the lung parenchyma, inflammation and oxidative stress, which plays a key role in the pathogenesis of the disease [Di Rosanna P et al., 2012; Alqahtani JS, et al., 2020; Collins PF et al., 2012; Barnes PJ et al., 2003; Barnes PJ et al., 2016].

In addition to external risk factors, genetic predisposition also plays a significant role in the development of COPD [Adcock IM et al., 2011; Moll M et al., 2020; Kirkham PA et al., 2013; Hardin M et al., 2014]. Congenital alpha-1-antitrypsin deficiency (α1-AT) is one of the proven genetic risk factors for the development of COPD. Alpha-1-antitrypsin is a serine protease inhibitor and its main function is to inhibit neutrophil elastase. Its inadequate inhibition leads to destruction of the lung parenchyma and the subsequent development of emphysema (see [Stoller JK et al., 2005]). In patients with low alpha-1-antitrypsin levels, nicotine consumption has been shown to significantly reduce FEV1 [Seersholm N et al., 1995; Hiller AM et al., 2019].

From all the above, the interaction between genetic and environmental factors in the development and progression of COPD is crucial for the clinical picture of the disease. Smoking and air pollution are the main risk factors for the development of COPD. The most important air pollutants are nitrogen dioxide (NO_2), sulfur dioxide (SO_2), ozone (O_3) and exhaust particles [Kiros F et al., 2016; Afroz R et al., 2003]. Different individual susceptibility to lung parenchymal destruction caused by nicotine and air pollution is due to differences in the expression of the phenotype, which indicates the interaction of environmental factors and genetic factors in the development of COPD (Figure 1).

Note: The relationship between the severity of airflow limitation and health status is known to be statistically significant. However, the individual variability of this parameter is so great that it cannot be accurately predicted in a single patient using FEV1 values, according to the primary authors.

Source: [Agusti A et al., 2016, p. 30] (Figure 1)

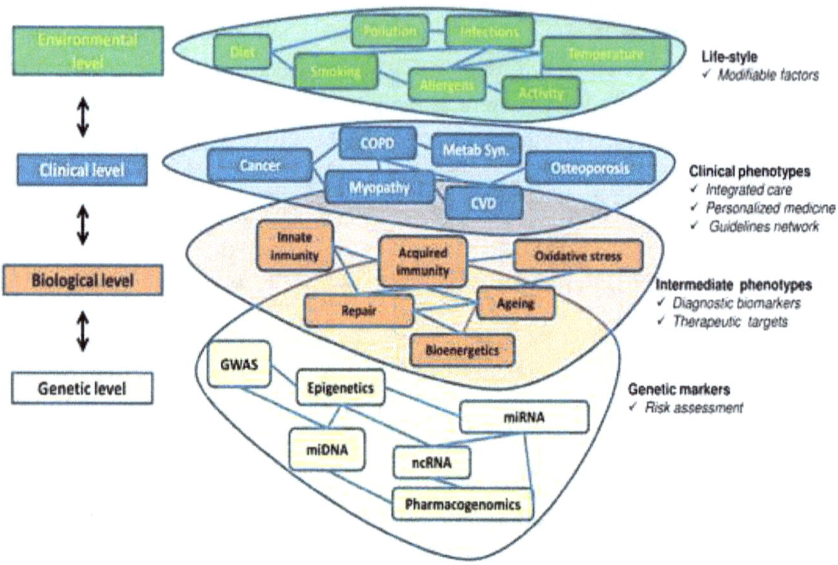

The interaction of the aforementioned factors activates various bio humoral mechanisms that alter genetic activity and lead to the development of endotypes that influence the expression of phenotypic characteristics. Identification of endotypes, by determining specific markers, is of clinical importance in the diagnosis and therapy of COPD.

1.3. Pathogenesis of Chronic Obstructive Pulmonary Disease

It is desirable, or rather necessary, to detect lung infection in the early phase of the disease. Early diagnosis and therapy, before the infection progresses to clinically significant inflammation and damage to the lung parenchyma, is of great importance and represents primary prevention [Bellamy D et al., 2007; Drummond MB et al., 2017; Sekine Y et al., 2012]. Pathological changes lead to air trapping in the airways. They also lead to progressive obstruction of airflow through the airways. Pathological changes generally occur in almost all structures of the lung tissue, in the airways as well as in the vascular network of the lungs. As a result, chronic inflammation develops, with numerous cells and other mediators of inflammation, which leads to structural changes in the lungs. According to studies by Rabe et al., Durstine et al., López-Campos et al., primary prevention is already being implemented in many countries and is expected to reduce the number of complications and consequences of pulmonary obstruction in the long term. It is also expected to reduce the transmission and spread of infection in the population and therefore reduce the incidence and associated sequelae (secondary prevention) [Rabe KF et al., 2007; Durstine JL et al., 2013; López-Campos JL et al., 2016].

The pathophysiological disorders and clinical manifestations of COPD are the result of the action of various factors and pathological disorders in the lungs [Belvisi MG et al., 2003; Baraldo S et al., 2012; Eapen MS et al., 2018]. The harmful effects of lung infection can be reduced through primary and secondary prevention, but they largely depend on the natural course of the infection.

1.4. Clinical Manifestations (Symptoms and Diagnoses) and Complications of Chronic Obstructive Pulmonary Disease

Initially, the basic symptoms and signs of chronic obstructive pulmonary disease develop slowly. The most common symptom is shortness of breath, which sufferers describe as shortness of breath, followed by a productive cough. As the disease progresses, normal daily activities become more difficult. Sufferers report that climbing a small number of stairs or carrying light loads becomes increasingly difficult. However, these symptoms may not occur until significant lung damage occurs, especially if the patient continues to be exposed to risk factors [Cohen BH et al., 1977; Brashier BB et al., 2012; GOLD, 2023].

Other symptoms of this disease include shortness of breath, especially on exertion, wheezing, chest tightness, morning sputum production, chronic cough, cyanosis of the lips, frequent respiratory infections, fatigue, and unintentional weight loss. As the disease progresses, symptoms related to chronic respiratory failure and chronic core pulmonale develop, which characterizes the terminal phase of the disease. All of these symptoms can vary, which must be considered when diagnosing [Čekerevac I, 2010; Jelić I et al., 2023; GOLD, 2023; Trivić B, 2016].

COPD is now considered a disease characterized not only by pulmonary but also by systemic inflammation. Systemic inflammation is the cause of numerous extrapulmonary manifestations. These systemic effects include cardiovascular disease, lung cancer, osteoporosis, anemia, gastroesophageal reflux, malnutrition, muscle weakness, and depression. All these diseases contribute significantly to the morbidity and mortality of COPD patients.

1.4.1. Symptoms and Diagnosis

The clinical diagnosis of COPD is based on symptoms such as dyspnea, chronic cough, sputum production, exposure to risk factors, and spirometry.

Severity assessment based on spirometry

COPD is classified into four stages according to the GOLD criteria [GOLD, 2023], according to the values of forced expiratory volume in the first second – FEV1 (Table 2).

Table 2. COPD disease stages, FEV1 reference values

GOLD 1 (Stage I)	Mild	FEV1 $\geq$ 80%
GOLD 2 (Stage II)	Moderate	FEV1 from 50% to 80%
GOLD 3 (Stage III)	Severe	FEV1 from 30% to 50%
GOLD 4 (Stage IV)	Very severe	FEV1 $\leq$ 30%

Source: Adapted from [GOLD, 2023, p. 37]

In relation to FEV1, there is mild, moderate, severe and very severe COPD. FEV1 values >80% characterize mild, 50-80% moderate, 30-50% severe and <30% very severe COPD.

A large number of studies have shown that in addition to pulmonary indicators, there are other factors that are important for assessing the severity of the disease, and to a large extent influence the prognosis and survival of COPD patients. These factors include: nutritional status, metabolic parameters, percentage of total body mass in the body (body fat percentage, FAT or BF), functional capacity, the ability of patients to exercise, implementation of physical treatment, the presence and number of associated diseases, i.e. comorbidities, etc. [Liu D et al., 2020; Furutate R et al., 2016; Graumam RQ et al., 2018].

In the 2018 revision of GOLD, new indicators were introduced for assessing disease severity in daily work, including: symptom assessment, assessment of the risk of acute exacerbations and assessment of comorbidities. These indicators provide better insight into the assessment of the impact of the disease on the health status and quality of life of the patient. They can be used to predict the risk of future adverse events, exacerbations, hospitalization and mortality. They do not exclude the assessment of disease severity based on FEV1, but complement and confirm it [GOLD, 2018; Ministarstvo zdravlja Republike Srbije, 2011].

Assessment of dyspnea

When it comes to assessing dyspnea, GOLD recommends using the Modified British Medical Research Council (mMRC) dyspnea scale (Table 3) [GOLD, 2023].

Table 3. Modified Medical Research Council Dyspnea Scale for COPD (mMRC scale), 0-4

Level 0	Shortness of breath only during strenuous exercise
Level 1	Shortness of breath during rapid walking (rushing) at walking level or slightly uphill
Level 2	Slower walking on level ground in people of the same age due to shortness of breath or needing to stop to catch one's breath when walking at one's own pace on level ground
Level 3	Stopping to catch your breath after walking about 100 meters or after a few minutes of walking on level ground
Level 4	Excessive shortness of breath when going out, i.e. leaving the house, or excessive shortness of breath when getting dressed or undressed

Source: [GOLD, 2023]

COPD is often associated with other diseases that can have a significant impact on the outcome of the disease. Some of them are independent of COPD, while others may be related to the causative agents of the disease or because one disease increases the risk of another disease. The reason for this is that due to systemic inflammation in COPD, extrapulmonary disorders exist, and smoking, as a common risk factor for many associated diseases (cardiovascular disease, anemia, osteoporosis, anxiety, depression, and other diseases), has a negative effect and increases the possibility of comorbidity [Zareifopoulos N et al, 2019; Dua R et al., 2018; Crisafulli E et al., 2008: Yin HL et al., 2017; van den Bemt L et al., 2009; Cavaillès A et al., 2013; Martinez CH et al., 2014].

Comorbidities occur at all stages of COPD and are independent predictors of hospitalization and mortality. They contribute greatly to the patients' health-related quality of life. Due to the frequency and importance of comorbidities in the diagnosis of COPD, they need to be sought. On the other hand, even when a present or possible comorbidity is diagnosed, it is necessary to search for COPD, if risk factors are present. It is especially important to pay attention to smoking and genetic predisposition [Zhou X et al., 2012; Marsh S et al., 2006; Yoshida T et al., 2007; Hardin M et al., 2014; Wagena E et al., 2004; Burney P et al., 2014; Loi AT et al., 2013].

It is estimated that about 10-40% of patients with somatic complaints also have a depressive disorder [Mohit MA et al., 2011; Adibi P et al., 2016]. According to WHO forecasts and the established increased rate of depression, experts indicate that by 2030 depression will be the most common cause of morbidity in the world [Lépine JP et al., 2011; WHO, 2004].

Results from a French study indicate that 41% of patients with chronic illness either have severe depression or, in most cases, it was unrecognized and untreated, and in only 6% of cases psychiatric help was sought [Fuhrer R et al., 1995]. Comorbid depression may be responsible for psychological mechanisms related to the patient's and social perception of the illness [Maurer J et al., 2008; Gatchel RJ, 2004; Markowitz S et al., 2008], but it may also be related to the etiological connection between somatic and psychological illness [Cougle JR et al., 2010; Katz IR, 1996; Batstra L et al., 2002; Liu Y et al., 2018].

---

[1]*GOLD. Global Strategy for the Diagnosis, Management and Prevention of Chronic Obstructive Pulmonary Disease: 2021 Report. 2021. Available https://goldcopd.org/wp-content/uploads/2020/11/GOLD-REPORT-2021-v1.1-25Nov20_WMV.pdf. Accessed: July 26, 2021.*
[2]*Hogea SP, Tudorache E, Fildan AP, Fira-Mladinescu O, Marc M, Oancea C. Risk factors of chronic obstructive pulmonary disease exacerbations. Clin Respir J. 2020;14(3):183–197. doi:10.1111/crj.13129.*
[3]*AIHW. Chronic Obstructive Pulmonary Disease (COPD). Cat. No. ACM 35. (Australian Institute of Health and Welfare, 2020).*

[4]Lazic Z, Stankovic I, Milenkovic B, Zvezdin B, Hromis S, Jankovic S, et al. Characteristics of COPD Phenotypes in Serbia. Int J Chron Obstruct Pulmon Dis. 2021;16:643-54.

[5]WHO. Chronic obstructive pulmonary disease (COPD). Available at https://www.who.int/news-room/fact-sheets/detail/chronic-obstructive-pulmonary-disease-(copd) Published June 21, 2021. Accessed: July 24, 2021.

[6]GOLD. Global strategyfor the diagnosis, management, and prevention of chronic obstructive pulmonarydisease. Updated 2018, 2018. http://www.goldcopd.org. https://goldcopd.org/wp-content/uploads/2017/11/GOLD-2018-v6.0-FINAL-revised-20-Nov_WMS.pdf

[7]Zareifopoulos N, Bellou A, Spiropoulou A, Spiropoulos K. Prevalence, contribution to disease burden and management of comorbid depression and anxiety in chronic obstructive pulmonary disease: a narrative review. COPD J Chronic Obstr Pulm Dis. 2019;16(5–6):406–417. doi:10.1080/15412555.2019.1679102

[8]Dua R, Das A, Kumar A, Kumar S, Mishra M, Sharma K. Association of comorbid anxiety and depression with chronic obstructive pulmonary disease. Lung India 2018;35:31-6.

[9]Wang J, Willis K, Barson E, Smallwood N. The complexity of mental health care for people with COPD: a qualitative study of clinicians' perspectives. NPJ primary care respiratory medicine. 2021 Jul 22;31(1):40.

[10]GOLD. Global Strategy for the Diagnosis, Management and Prevention of Chronic Obstructive Pulmonary Disease: 2019 Report, 2019. www.goldcopd.org (Accessed on February 04, 2019).

[11]Wrzeciono A, Czech O, Buchta K, Zabłotni S, Gos E, Tłuczykont Ł, Górecka D, Pastuła A, Adamczyk M, Jach E, Świerkowski I. Assessment of stress, depressive and anxiety symptoms in patients with COPD during in-hospital pulmonary rehabilitation: an observational cohort study. Medicina. 2021 Feb 25;57(3):197.

[12]Rosińczuk J, Przyszlak M, Uchmanowicz I. Sociodemographic and clinical factors affecting the quality of life of patients with chronic obstructive pulmonary disease. International journal of chronic obstructive pulmonary disease. 2018 Sep 12:2869-82. doi: 10.2147/COPD.S165714

[13]Safiri S, Carson-Chahhoud K, Noori M, Nejadghaderi SA, Sullman MJ, Heris JA, Ansarin K, Mansournia MA, Collins GS, Kolahi AA, Kaufman JS. Burden of chronic obstructive pulmonary disease and its attributable risk factors in 204 countries and territories, 1990-2019: results from the Global Burden of Disease Study 2019. bmj. 2022 Jul 27;378.

[14]*Batut. Institut za javno zdravlje Srbije „Dr Milan Jovanović Batut“, Zdravstveno statistički godišnjak. Studija „Istraživanje zdravlja stanovništva Srbije 2019. godine”; 2019. https://www.batut.org.rs/download/publikacije/ZdravljeStanovnistva2019.pdf*

[15]*Batut. Здравствено-статистички годишњак Републике Србије 2021, 2021. https://www.batut.org.rs/download/publikacije/pub2021a.pdf*

[16]*Vukoja M, Kopitovic I, Lazic, Z, Milenkovic B, Stankovic I, Zvezdin B et al. Diagnosis and management of chronic obstructive pulmonary disease in Serbia: an expert group position statement. Int J Chron Obstruct Pulmon Dis. 2019; 14: 1993–2002.*

[17]*Pejčić T. Definicija i epidemiologija opstruktivne bolesti pluća. U: Bošnjak-Petrović B,ured Hronična opstruktivna bolest pluća. Beograd: Libri medicorum, 2011.*

[18]*Milenković B, Mitić-Milikić M, Rebić P, Vukčević M, Dudvarski-Ilić A, NagorniObradović Lj, Lazić Z, Bošnjak-Petrović V. Asthma and Chronic Bronchitis Symptomsamong Adult Population of Belgrade. Srp Arh CelokLek2011;139(3-4)149-154*

[19]*Stanković I. Faktori rizika za nastanak hronične opstruktivne bolesti pluća. U: BošnjakPetrović V. Hronična opstruktivna bolest pluća. Beograd: Libri medicorum, 2011.*

[20]*Čekerevac I. Sistemski efekti hronične opstruktivne bolesti pluća. Doktorska disertacija, Kragujevac, 2010.*

[21]*Ivana Jelić, Goran Mihajlović, Miloš Ratinac, Katarina Mihajlović, Sara Mijailović and Ivan Cekerevac, Psychophysical and Social Functioning of Patients with Chronic Obstructive Lung Disease and Depression, Eur. J. Investig. Health Psychol. Educ. 2023, 13, 2841–2852. https://doi.org/10.3390/ejihpe13120196.*

[22]*Bošnjak-Petrović V. Sistemski efekti i komorbiditet u hroničnoj opstruktivnoj bolesti pluća. U: Bošnjak-Petrović V. Hronična opstruktivna bolest pluća. Beograd: Libri medicorum, 2011, стр. 251-68.*

[23]*GOLD. (2013). Global Initiative for Chronic Obstructive Lung Disease (GOLD) 2013. http://www.goldcopd.org/.*

[24]*Antuni JD, Barnes PJ. Evaluation of individuals at risk for COPD: beyond the scope of the global initiative for chronic obstructive lung disease. Chronic Obstructive Pulmonary Diseases: Journal of the COPD Foundation. 2016;3(3):653.*

[25]Zhou X, Baron RM, Hardin M, et al. Identification of a chronic obstructive pulmonary disease genetic determinant that regulates HHIP. Hum Mol Genet 2012; 21:1325.
[26]Dome P, Lazary J, Kalapos MP, Rihmer Z. Smoking, nicotine and neuropsychiatric disorders. Neuroscience & Biobehavioral Reviews. 2010 Feb 1;34(3):295-342.
[27]U.S. Department of Health and Human Services. The Health Consequences of Smoking— 50 Years of Progress: A Report of the Surgeon General. Atlanta: U.S. Department of Health and Human Services, Centers for Disease Control and Prevention, National Center for Chronic Disease Prevention and Health Promotion, Office on Smoking and Health, 2014.
[28]Marsh S, Aldington S, Shirtcliffe P, Weatherall M, Beasley R. Smoking and COPD: what really are the risks? Eur. Respir. J. 2006; 28:883–886.
[29]Hikichi M, Mizumura K, Maruoka S, Gon Y. Pathogenesis of chronic obstructive pulmonary disease (COPD) induced by cigarette smoke. Journal of thoracic disease. 2019 Oct;11(Suppl 17):S2129.
[30]Lamprecht B, McBurnie MA, Vollmer WM, et al. COPD in never smokers: results from the population-based burden of obstructive lung disease study. Chest, 2011; 139(4):752-63.
[31]Di Rosanna P, Salvatore C. Reactive oxygen species, inflammation, and lung diseases. Current pharmaceutical design. 2012 Sep 1;18(26):3889-900.
[32]Benowitz NL, Hatsukami D. Gender differences in the pharmacology of nicotine addiction. Addiction biology. 1998 Oct;3(4):383-404.
[33]Yoshida T, Tuder RM. Pathobiology of cigarette smoke-induced chronic obstructive pulmonary disease. Physiological reviews. 2007 Jul;87(3):1047-82.
[34]Jain D, Chaudhary P, Varshney N, Bin Razzak KS, Verma D, Khan Zahra TR, Janmeda P, Sharifi-Rad J, Daştan SD, Mahmud S, Docea AO. Tobacco smoking and liver cancer risk: potential avenues for carcinogenesis. Journal of Oncology. 2021 Dec 10;2021.
[35]Alqahtani JS, Njoku CM, Bereznicki B, Wimmer BC, Peterson GM, Kinsman L, Aldabayan YS, Alrajeh AM, Aldhahir AM, Mandal S, Hurst JR. Risk factors for all-cause hospital readmission following exacerbation of COPD: a systematic review and meta-analysis. Eur Respir Rev. 2020 Jun 3;29(156):190166. doi: 10.1183/16000617.0166-2019. PMID: 32499306.
[36]Collins PF, Stratton RJ, Elia M. Nutritional support in chronic obstructive pulmonary disease: a systematic review and meta-analysis. Am J Clin Nutr. 2012; 95:1385–1395. 76.

[37]*Barnes PJ, Shapiro SD, Pauwels RA. Chronic obstructive pulmonary disease: molecular and cellular mechanisms. European Respiratory Journal. 2003 Oct 1;22(4):672-88.*

[38]*Barnes PJ. Inflammatory mechanisms in patients with chronic obstructive pulmonary disease. Journal of Allergy and Clinical Immunology. 2016 Jul 1;138(1):16-27.*

[39]*Adcock IM, Caramori G, Barnes PJ. Chronic obstructive pulmonary disease and lung cancer: new molecular insights. Respiration. 2011;81(4):265-84.*

[40]*Moll M, Sakornsakolpat P, Shrine N, Hobbs BD, DeMeo DL, John C, Guyatt AL, McGeachie MJ, Gharib SA, Obeidat ME, Lahousse L. Chronic obstructive pulmonary disease and related phenotypes: polygenic risk scores in population-based and case-control cohorts. The Lancet Respiratory Medicine. 2020 Jul 1;8(7):696-708.*

[41]*Kirkham PA, Barnes PJ. Oxidative stress in COPD. Chest. 2013 Jul 1;144(1):266-73.*

[42]*Hardin M, Silverman EK. Chronic obstructive pulmonary disease genetics: a review of the past and a look into the future. Chronic Obstructive Pulmonary Diseases: Journal of the COPD Foundation. 2014;1(1):33.*

[43]*Stoller JK, Aboussouan LS. Alpha1-antitrypsin deficiency. Lancet. 2005; 365(9478):2225-36.*

[44]*Seersholm N, Kok-Jensen A, Dirksen A. Decline in FEV1 among patients with severe hereditary alpha 1-antitrypsin deficiency type PiZ. American journal of respiratory and critical care medicine. 1995 Dec;152(6):1922-5.*

[45]*Hiller AM, Piitulainen E, Jehpsson L, Tanash H. Decline in FEV1 and hospitalized exacerbations in individuals with severe alpha-1 antitrypsin deficiency. International journal of chronic obstructive pulmonary disease. 2019 May 23:1075-83.*

[46]*Kiros F, Shakya KM, Rupakheti M, Regmi RP, Maharjan R, Byanju RM, Naja M, Mahata K, Kathayat B, Peltier RE. Variability of anthropogenic gases: Nitrogen oxides, sulfur dioxide, ozone and ammonia in Kathmandu Valley, Nepal. Aerosol and Air Quality Research. 2016 Dec;16(12):3088-101.*

[47]*Afroz R, Hassan MN, Ibrahim NA. Review of air pollution and health impacts in Malaysia. Environmental research. 2003 Jun 1;92(2):71-7.*

[48]*Agusti A, Gea J, Faner R. Biomarkers, the control panel and personalized COPD medicine. Respirology. 2016 Jan;21(1):24-33.*

[49]*Bellamy D, Smith J. Role of primary care in early diagnosis and effective management of COPD. International journal of clinical practice. 2007 Aug;61(8):1380-9.*
[50]*Drummond MB, Buist AS, Crapo JD, Wise RA, Rennard SI. Chronic obstructive pulmonary disease: NHLBI workshop on the primary prevention of chronic lung diseases. Annals of the American Thoracic Society. 2014 Apr;11(Supplement 3):S154-60.*
[51]*Sekine Y, Katsura H, Koh E, Hiroshima K, Fujisawa T. Early detection of COPD is important for lung cancer surveillance. European Respiratory Journal. 2012 May 1;39(5):1230-40.*
[52]*Rabe KF, Hurd S, Anzueto A, Barnes PJ, Buist SA, Calverley P, Fukuchi Y, Jenkins C, Rodriguez-Roisin R, Van Weel C, Zielinski J. Global strategy for the diagnosis, management, and prevention of chronic obstructive pulmonary disease: GOLD executive summary. American journal of respiratory and critical care medicine. 2007 Sep 15;176(6):532-55.*
[53]*Durstine JL, Gordon B, Wang Z, Luo X. Chronic disease and the link to physical activity. Journal of sport and health science. 2013 Mar 1;2(1):3-11.*
[54]*López-Campos JL, Tan W, Soriano JB. Global burden of COPD. Respirology. 2016 Jan;21(1):14-23.*
[55]*Belvisi MG, Bottomley KM. The role of matrix metalloproteinases (MMPs) in the pathophysiology of chronic obstructive pulmonary disease (COPD): a therapeutic role for inhibitors of MMPs?. Inflammation research. 2003 Mar;52:95-100.*
[56]*Baraldo S, Turato G, Saetta M. Pathophysiology of the small airways in chronic obstructive pulmonary disease. Respiration. 2012;84(2):89-97.*
[57]*Eapen MS, Hansbro PM, Larsson-Callerfelt AK, Jolly MK, Myers S, Sharma P, Jones B, Rahman MA, Markos J, Chia C, Larby J. Chronic obstructive pulmonary disease and lung cancer: underlying pathophysiology and new therapeutic modalities. Drugs. 2018 Nov;78:1717-40.*
[58]*Wilkinson TM, Aris E, Bourne S, Clarke SC, Peeters M, Pascal TG, Schoonbroodt S, Tuck AC, Kim V, Ostridge K, Staples KJ. A prospective, observational cohort study of the seasonal dynamics of airway pathogens in the aetiology of exacerbations in COPD. Thorax. 2017 Oct 1;72(10):919-27.*
[59]*Batut. Nacionalni vodič dobre kliničke prakse za dijagnostiku i lečenje Hronične opstruktivne bolesti pluća. 2013. https://www.batut.org.rs/download/aktuelno/klinicka%20praksa/Hronicna%20opstruktivna%20bolest%20pluca.pdf*

[60]*Chung KF, Adcock IM. Multifaceted mechanisms in COPD: inflammation, immunity, and tissue repair and destruction. European Respiratory Journal. 2008 Jun 1;31(6):1334-56.*
[61]*Zhou Y, Fu B, Zheng X, Wang D, Zhao C, Qi Y, Sun R, Tian Z, Xu X, Wei H. Aberrant pathogenic GM-CSF+ T cells and inflammatory CD14+ CD16+ monocytes in severe pulmonary syndrome patients of a new coronavirus. biorxiv. 2020 Feb 20:2020-02.*
[62]*Azkur AK, Akdis M, Azkur D, Sokolowska M, van de Veen W, Brüggen MC, O'Mahony L, Gao Y, Nadeau K, Akdis CA. Immune response to SARS-CoV-2 and mechanisms of immunopathological changes in COVID-19. Allergy. 2020 Jul;75(7):1564-81.*
[63]*Vasiljević S. Socijalna dimenzija kvaliteta života obolelih od hronične opstruktivne bolesti pluća. Универзитет у Крагујевцу. 2019.*
Glencross DA, Ho TR, Camina N, Hawrylowicz CM, Pfeffer PE. Air pollution and its effects on the immune system. Free Radical Biology and Medicine. 2020 May 1;151:56-68.
[64]*Sharma, G., Hanania, N. A., & Shim, Y. M. (2009). The aging immune system and its relationship to the development of chronic obstructive pulmonary disease. Proceedings of the American Thoracic Society, 6(7), 573-580.*
[65]*Strzelak A, Ratajczak A, Adamiec A, Feleszko W. Tobacco smoke induces and alters immune responses in the lung triggering inflammation, allergy, asthma and other lung diseases: a mechanistic review. International journal of environmental research and public health. 2018 May;15(5):1033.*
[66]*Xue W, Ma J, Li Y, Xie C. Role of CD4+ T and CD8+ T Lymphocytes-Mediated Cellular Immunity in Pathogenesis of Chronic Obstructive Pulmonary Disease. Journal of Immunology Research. 2022;2022.*
Brusselle GG, Joos GF, Bracke KR. New insights into the immunology of chronic obstructive pulmonary disease. The Lancet. 2011 Sep 10;378(9795):1015-26.
[67]*Gouwy M, Struyf S, Proost P, Van Damme J. Synergy in cytokine and chemokine networks amplifies the inflammatory response. Cytokine & growth factor reviews. 2005 Dec 1;16(6):561-80.*
[68]*Rovina N, Koutsoukou A, Koulouris NG. Inflammation and immune response in COPD: where do we stand?. Mediators of inflammation. 2013 Oct;2013.*
[69]*Cohen BH, BALL JR WC, Brashears S, Diamond EL, Kreiss P, Levy DA, Menkes HA, Permutt S, Tockman MS. Risk factors in chronic obstructive*

pulmonary disease (COPD). American journal of epidemiology. 1977 Mar 1;105(3):223-32.

[70]*Brashier BB, Kodgule R. Risk factors and pathophysiology of chronic obstructive pulmonary disease (COPD). J Assoc Physicians India. 2012 Feb 1;60(Suppl):17-21.*

[71]*GOLD. Global Initiative For Chronic Obstructive Lung Diseases. 2023 Report. 2023. https://goldcopd.org/2023-gold-report-2/*

[72]*Trivić B. Analiza troškova nastalih hospitalizacijom u tercijarnoj ustanovi usled akutnih egzacerbacija hronične opstruktivne bolesti pluća. Универзитет у Новом Саду. 2016 May 23.*

[73]*Liu D, Meister M, Zhang S, Vong CI, Wang S, Fang R, Li L, Wang PG, Massion P, Ji X. Identification of lipid biomarker from serum in patients with chronic obstructive pulmonary disease. Respiratory Research. 2020 Dec;21:1-3.*

[74]*Furutate R, Ishii T, Motegi T, Hattori K, Kusunoki Y, Gemma A, Kida K. The neutrophil to lymphocyte ratio is related to disease severity and exacerbation in patients with chronic obstructive pulmonary disease. Internal Medicine. 2016;55(3):223-9.*

[75]*Graumam RQ, Pinheiro MM, Nery LE, Castro CH. Increased rate of osteoporosis, low lean mass, and fragility fractures in COPD patients: association with disease severity. Osteoporosis International. 2018 Jun;29:1457-68.*

[76]*Ministarstvo zdravlja Republike Srbije. 2011. Национални водич добре клиничке праксе. Депресија. https://www.zdravlje.gov.rs/view_file.php?file_id=675&cache=sr;*

Mahler DA, Wells CK. Evaluation of clinical methods for rating dyspnea. Chest 1988; 93: 580–586.

[77]*Bestall JC, Paul EA, Garrod R, et al. Usefulness of the medical research council (MRC) dyspnoea scale as a measure of disability in patients with chronic obstructive pulmonary disease. Thorax 1999; 54: 581–586.*

[78]*Crisafulli E, Costi S, Luppi F, Cirelli G, Cilione C, Coletti O, Fabbri LM, Clini EM. Role of comorbidities in a cohort of patients with COPD undergoing pulmonary rehabilitation. Thorax. 2008 Jun 1;63(6):487-92.*

Yin HL, Yin SQ, Lin QY, Xu Y, Xu HW, Liu T. Prevalence of comorbidities in chronic obstructive pulmonary disease patients: a meta-analysis. Medicine. 2017 May;96(19).

[79]*van den Bemt L, Schermer T, Bor H, Smink R, van Weel-Baumgarten E, Lucassen P, van Weel C. The risk for depression comorbidity in patients with COPD. Chest. 2009 Jan 1;135(1):108-14.*

[80]Cavaillès A, Brinchault-Rabin G, Dixmier A et al. Comorbidities of COPD. Eur Resp Rev. 2013; 22: 454-475; doi: 10.1183/09059180.00008612
[81]Martinez CH, Mannino DM, Divo MJ. Defining COPD-related comorbidities, 2004-2014. J COPD F. 2014; 1(1): 51-63.
[82]Wagena Ej, Kant I, van Amelsvoort LG, et al. Risk of depression and anxiety in employees with chronic bronchitis: the modifying effect of cigarette smoking. Psychosom Med. 2004;66:729-734.
[83]Burney P, Jithoo A, Koto B, et al. Chronic obstructive pulmonary disease mortality and prevalence: the associations with smoking and poverty-a BOLD analysis. Thorax 2014; 69(5):465-473. 17.
[84]Loi AT, Hoonhorst SJ, Franciosi L, Bischoff R, Hoffmann RF, Heijink I, van Oosterhout AJ, Boezen HM, Timens W, Postma DS, Lammers JW. Acute and chronic inflammatory responses induced by smoking in individuals susceptible and non-susceptible to development of COPD: from specific disease phenotyping towards novel therapy. Protocol of a cross-sectional study. Bmj Open. 2013 Jan 1;3(2):e002178.

PART TWO

Depression – What Do You Need to Know?

2. Depression – Definition, Epidemiology, Symptoms, Diagnosis: What You Need to Know

Depression is often unrecognized or undertreated in patients with COPD [Lacasse Y et al., 2001; Wong TS et al., 2014; Yao HM et al., 2020; Kim KU et al., 2014; Lou P et al., 2014]. It ranges from short-term depressive episodes to clinically overt depression. Several studies have found that two-thirds of patients with COPD have moderate to severe depression (see [Maurer J et al., 2008; Katon W et al., 2002; Fritzsche A et al., 2011]. In a 2008 study by Maurer et al., it was reported that about one-quarter of COPD patients had unrecognized depression [Maurer J et al., 2008].

The impact of depression is significant not only for patients, but also for their families and communities [Billings AG et al., 1983; Brown J et al., 1999; Maharaj S et al., 2019; Solé B et al., 2021]. Depressed patients with chronic diseases are usually "sicker" than those without chronic diseases [LaGran B et al., 2020; Gray C et al., 2023].

Depression in COPD reduces quality of life [Balcells E. et al., 2010; Sundh J. et al., 2011; Pedrozo-Pupo J.C. et al., 2021]. Results from the National Emphysema Treatment Trial (NETT) indicate that depression increases the total number of hospitalizations and mortality in patients over a three-year period [Fan V.S. et al., 2007].

With treatment of COPD exacerbations, symptoms of depression spontaneously resolve in many patients' withdrawal. The main principles of treatment are antidepressants and psychotherapy [Jelić I et al., 2023, Cafarella PA et al., 2012; Yohannes AM et al., 2011; Lin P et al., 2005]. Selective serotonin reuptake inhibitors, as well as low-dose benzodiazepines, are the basis of drug therapy for depression in patients with COPD [Yohannes AM et al., 2022; Yohannes AM et al., 2017; Tselebis A et al., 2016]. In patients with respiratory failure, it is advisable to avoid sedative drugs [Zuo M et al., 2019; Chanques G et al., 2020]. Psychotherapy is an ideal treatment option for chronic patients who are already taking many medications [Keller MB et al., 2000; von Wietersheim J et al., 2006; Hamilton J et al., 2000; Nemeroff CB et al., 2003; Schramm E et al., 2019]. Less than 50% of patients with depression are recognized, which indicates the need for identification of patients in primary health care. A simple and quick way to detect symptoms of depression is the use of an adequate questionnaire [Urtasun M et al., 2019; Jelić I et al., 2013; Story DA et al., 2019; Morin A, 2021; APA,

2023; Ayalon L et al., 2010; Manea L et al., 2012], which will be discussed later in our book.

Symptoms of depression appear as early as the diagnosis of a chronic illness, accompanied by progressive impairment of physical function and a decrease in quality of life. Low mood, sleep disturbances, loss of appetite, fatigue, and cognitive impairment are some of the symptoms of depression that overlap with many other chronic illnesses. Loss of will to live and thoughts about the end of life are symptoms of depression that should be taken seriously and treated urgently.

2.1. The Definition of Depression

It is increasingly clear that mood disorders are the most common health conditions. These disorders have a high comorbidity potential. According to the International Classification of Diseases, version 10 (ICD-10) [Ministarstvo zdravlja Republike Srbije, 2011], these disorders are divided into:

- depressive episode (of varying degree and quality - with “somatic symptoms”, with “psychotic symptoms”),

- recurrent depressive disorder, which involves two depressive episodes separated by a symptom-free interval of 2 months, and

- persistent depressive disorder - dysthymia.

In depression, as in other mood disorders, not only is a mood disorder present, but other disorders of psychological function are also present [Ministarstvo zdravlja Republike Srbije, 2011; Peterson JB, 2002]. For example, in emotional disorders, a depressed mood is present, up to a feeling of unexplained sadness. It is very common for the person speaking to experience a transfer of emotions, or an empathetic experience of sadness, when in contact with a person suffering from depression. In deeper stages of depression, anhedonia is present, which means that the depressed person is unable to feel any pleasure or interest in their surroundings. When a depressed person is unable to rejoice, make decisions, or experience love, this is called Lehmann’s triad. Irritability and anxiety are often present in depression. In addition, depressed people are characterized by a dominant sense of guilt and worthlessness. When a depressed person negatively interprets the past and experiences, themselves, and future expectations, this is called Beck's triad. A thought disorder is also generally present, which is diagnosed by noticing that the thought process is extremely slowed down, even stopped. In other words, it takes a depressed person a long time to, for example, answer a question.

People with depression tend to exaggerate their own inabilities and catastrophe past, present, and future experiences. They are dissatisfied with their appearance, intellect, and life in general. A high level of dissatisfaction leads to a distortion of reality and even to delusional ideas of various forms. All this makes the person feel even more depressed, and in this way the depression deepens, and a "dry form" of depression can occur (the depressed person is no longer able to cry), which is a serious diagnostic sign.

In addition to emotions and thoughts, depression is often accompanied by other disorders of mental functions (attention, perception, memory, drives, will). In attention disorders, it is noticeable that a person has difficulty concentrating on any topic except the topics of worthlessness, guilt, and sadness. Under the strong influence of concentration on these topics, a person can recall distorted images from the past, which are characteristic of memory disorders. Depressed people can distort memories so much, up to the level of hallucinations, which also leads to a disturbance of perception (for example, they may feel that other people are talking about how guilty and sinful they are). As a result of these disorders, the drives to live, have sex, sleep, and eat can be significantly reduced. Long-term and deep depression leads to a loss of will (disorder of will), which is diagnosed by the person being noticeably without energy, ineffective in daily activities, and isolating themselves from everything and everyone. The loss of all will is called abulia.

Although they are classified in the group of mood disorders (affective disorders), in ICD-10 there is a clear division between depressive disorders, which are manifested only by symptoms belonging to the group of depressive syndromes (also called unipolar depressions), and bipolar disorders, which are manifested by manic/hypomanic states and depressive episodes. Depressive disorders, i.e. unipolar depression, are represented by psychological, behavioral and somatovegetative symptoms (Table 4).

Table 4. Symptoms of unipolar depression

Psychological	Behavioral	Somatovegetative
sorrow	withdrawal	fatigue
apathy	unconcern for the environment	sleep disorder
irritability	social distancing	appetite disorder
concentration disorder	physical inactivity	digestive problems
despair	lack of motivation	

Unipolar depressive disorder is a disorder in which the illness is characterized exclusively by depressive episodes. When these episodes recur, it is called recurrent depressive disorder [Ministarstvo zdravlja i socijalne zaštite Republike Srpske, 2008].

Although depression can occur only once in a lifetime, people can experience multiple depressive episodes. Symptoms of depression are usually present for most of the day. They include feelings of sadness, anger, and emptiness [Peterson JB, 2002]. Some of the other symptoms include sleep disturbances, decreased activity, and anxiety. Sleep disturbances can cause a person to sleep too much or be too tired and can affect or be related to a person's weight and appetite. Decreased physical activity and weight loss can also be symptoms of depression. Compulsions or anxiety can cause a person to feel guilty or worthless, and together with other factors, can trigger thoughts of suicide or self-blame.

Symptoms of depression can be severe enough to cause people to feel unhappy or miserable at work, school, or in social situations [Peterson JB, 2002]. Some individuals may not know why they feel this way, which is why diagnosis and subsequent treatment (psychotherapy, cognitive-behavioral therapy, and/or medication) play a key role in recovering from a depressive episode or depressive state.

2.2. Epidemiology

In collaboration with the WHO-WMH (World Mental Health Organization), a survey was conducted in developed and middle-income countries to estimate the global prevalence of depression. The survey included 89000 people from 18 countries. The results showed that 15-28% of the population in developed countries has depression, and in middle-income countries 11-20%. High rates of depression have been observed in France (around 30%), the Netherlands and the United States, with the lowest incidence in China (12%) [Bromet E et al., 2011].

Data from studies suggest that depression is more common in females [Waraich P et al., 2004]. The prevalence of major depressive episodes among adolescents in the United States increased by 7.7% (from 8.1% to 15.8%) and among girls by 12% (from 11.4% to 23.4%) between 2009 and 2019. The gender gap in the prevalence of major depressive episodes in these countries increased from 6.4% to 14.8% over the same ten-year period [Daly M, 2022].

Given the epidemiological data and the numerous socioeconomic factors that significantly influence the prevalence rate, treatment of depression and the comorbidity of depression with chronic physical illnesses is of crucial importance [WHO, 2021; WHO, 2022].

2.2.1. Epidemiological Trends in Depression in the United States

The most reported mental illness in the United States is depression. The overall rate of depression in the United States is constantly increasing [Lépine JP et al., 2011; Baxter AJ et al., 2014; Greenberg PE et al., 2015].

In addition to the increased incidence of depressive symptoms, these epidemiological trends are also significantly influenced by using adequate questionnaires to assess depressive symptoms, as well as more complete reporting by institutions. The increased use of screening examinations in the last decade has increased the number of reported cases (see [O'Connor EA et al., 2010; Williams LJ et al., 2016; Siniscalchi KA et al., 2020]). Accordingly, the increase in the number of reported cases of depression may be influenced by an increase in incidence, the use of standardized questionnaires, screening examinations, and more complete reporting. Similarly, the decrease in the number of reported cases of depression may be influenced by a decrease in incidence or the number of screening examinations.

In 2018, a total of 1,698,355 cases were reported to the Centers for Disease Control, which means that the rate of depression was 498.4 cases per 100,000 population. Compared to 2017, this rate showed an increase of 4.8%. The increase was recorded in all parts of the United States in the period from 2017 to 2018, with the Northeast region reporting the highest rate of 9% [NCHC, 2023a; NCHC, 2023b; NCHC, 2023c; NCHC, 2023d].

2.2.2. Epidemiological Trends in Depression in Europe

The overall prevalence of depression in Europe is high but stable [130-133]. Between 2016 and 2020, the number of cases reported to the European Centre for Disease Prevention and Control from 26 countries increased from 368,479 to 398,139, representing 197 cases per 100,000 population, but there is wide variation between countries and their reported rates [ECDC, 2023]. Countries reporting over 200 cases per 100,000 (e.g. Iceland, Norway, Sweden, United Kingdom) have well-implemented disease prevention and control programmers, based primarily on the recommendation of annual screening. The reporting rate is highest in younger women (240/100,000). In men, the reported rate is considerably lower (156/100,000) [ECDC, 2023].

There is wide variation across European countries in reported rates of depressive illness [Van de Velde S et al., 2010; Ibrahim AK et al., 2013; Arias-de la Torre J et al., 2021]. The very low rates in some Central and Eastern European countries may be due to changes in health systems and increased use of private practices that do not report to screening programs.

2.2.3. Epidemiological Trends in Depression in Serbia

The rate of depression in the Republic of Serbia is low, i.e. 5% of the total population. In addition to the low rate of reported cases, this epidemiological trend is significantly influenced by the diagnostic procedures used to diagnose depression, as well as reporting by institutions. Furthermore, visiting private practices, which do not report the results of screening examinations, also contributes to these trends. In the period from 2014 to 2017, there were no significant variations in the incidence of symptoms of depression. In 2017, 954 cases were reported, giving an incidence of 13.32%, in 2015, 941 cases were reported and an incidence of 13.19%, while in 2016, the incidence was slightly lower than the previous year and amounted to 12.65%, or 893 reported cases per total population. According to WHO estimates, 419,302 people in our country suffer from depression. Although it is a disease that is successfully treated in most cases, depression claims about 800,000 lives worldwide annually [WHO, 2017; Pravno informacioni sistem Republike Srbije, 2019; Martinović I, 2019; WHO, 2018].

Estimates by the authorities in Serbia indicate that about 1,300 people with depressive symptoms are killed every year, which places our country in 13th place in Europe [Ministarstvo zdravlja Republike Srbije, 2011; Martinović I, 2019]. Suicidal ideation is one of the symptoms of severe depression, and the suicide rate suggests that each of us knows someone who has committed suicide. Although the elderly population is generally more prone to suicide, according to data from the Institute of Public Health "Milan Jovanović Batut", the symptoms of depression are shifting towards the younger age [Batut, 2019; Batut, 2011].

2.3. Socioeconomic Consequences of the Disease

A decade ago, it was estimated that about 121 million people worldwide suffer from depression, and that about 850 thousand deaths occur due to depression every year [Ministarstvo zdravlja i socijalne zaštite Republike Srpske, 2008]. Therefore, depression should be recognized and treated in a timely manner. Depression leads to impaired psychosocial functioning. It also increases morbidity, mortality and the use of health services, which is largely reflected in the socio-economic aspect of this disorder both for the patient and their family, as well as society.

Work disability and impairment of psychosocial functioning of the sufferer are a major problem for the community and WHO data indicate that it will be in fourth place in the incidence of the disease [Bromet E et al., 2011; WHO, 2021].

The economic burden created by depression is, therefore, significant. The use of health care services by depressed patients is 50-100% higher compared to non-depressed patients [Jaffe DH et al., 2019; Greenberg PE et al., 2021; APA, 2021; Keshavarz K et al., 2022; Johnston KM et al., 2019].

2.4. Diagnosis of Depressive Disorders

Depression is more difficult to diagnose than somatic illnesses, because there are no laboratory tests that would confirm the presence of depressive illness. In addition, the symptoms of depression are numerous and diverse. They range from different forms of mood swings to somatovegetative complaints, they vary in severity from mild to severe, and manifest differently in the patient. Many patients present with somatic symptoms of depressive disorder, such as headaches, back pain, muscle weakness, and others, which overlap with symptoms of various somatic diseases [Ministarstvo zdravlja Republike Srbije, 2011; Ministarstvo zdravlja i socijalne zaštite Republike Srpske, 2008; Goldenberg DL, 2009; Kimmel PL et al., 1993].

The diagnosis of depression is based on the diagnostic criteria of the International Classification of Diseases, Tenth Revision (ICD-10). The first step in recognizing a depressive disorder is to diagnose a depressive episode. The diagnostic criteria for a depressive episode are the duration of symptoms of at least 2 weeks, typical symptoms of depressed mood, loss of interest and pleasure, decreased energy, increased fatigue, and decreased activity. Other symptoms may also be present, such as decreased concentration and attention, decreased self-esteem, feelings of guilt and worthlessness, a pessimistic view of the future, thoughts of self-harm or suicide, sleep disturbances, and decreased appetite [Ministarstvo zdravlja Republike Srbije, 2011; Ministarstvo zdravlja i socijalne zaštite Republike Srpske, 2008; Gruenberg AM et al., 2005; Löwe B et al., 2004; WHO, 1992].

To make a diagnosis of depression, it is necessary to conduct a diagnostic interview with the patient and observe the patient's behavior during the interview. It is desirable to obtain data from family members. In many countries, the use of diagnostic instruments (standardized questionnaires and scales) is also accepted [Ministarstvo zdravlja Republike Srbije, 2011; Ministarstvo zdravlja i socijalne zaštite Republike Srpske, 2008; Löwe B et al., 2004; WHO, 1992; Rizzo R et al., 2000].

To make a diagnosis of depressive disorder, it is necessary to exclude the existence of other psychiatric disorders. The diagnostic procedure includes not only taking detailed psychiatric history and evaluating mental status, but also a somatic and neurological examination, laboratory tests (complete blood count, biochemical blood and urine tests), endocrinological tests (especially thyroid function), as well as determining the presence/absence of psychoactive substances.

According to the ICD-10, there are three stages of depression:

I Mild depression,

II Moderate depression,

III Severe depression.

For the diagnosis of depression, symptoms are divided into two groups (group A and group B).

Group A contains three symptoms:

1. Depressed mood,
2. Loss of pleasure and interest,
3. Increased fatigue.

Group B contains 7 symptoms:

1. Loss of concentration (impaired attention),
2. Reduced self-esteem and self-confidence,
3. Feelings of worthlessness and guilt,
4. Pessimistic view of the future,
5. Ideas about self-harm and/or suicide,
6. Disturbed (decreased) appetite,
7. Disturbed (decreased or increased) sleep.

When a person has at least 2 out of 3 symptoms from group A and at least 2 out of 7 symptoms from group B, mild depression is diagnosed.

When a person has 2 out of 3 symptoms from group A and 3-4 out of 7 symptoms from group B, moderate depression is diagnosed.

When a person has 3 out of 3 symptoms from group A, 4 or more symptoms from group B and somatic syndrome of depression, severe depression is diagnosed.

Somatic syndrome of depression is diagnosed when a person has at least 4 out of 6 symptoms:

1. Early morning awakening,
2. Feeling worse in the morning,
3. Loss of libido,
4. Weight loss (at least 5% in a month),
5. Physical slowness or restlessness,
6. Anhedonia.

Somatic depression may also be present in mild to moderate depression. In this case, it is mild to moderate depression with somatic signs [Ministarstvo zdravlja i socijalne zaštite Republike Srpske, 2008; WHO, 1992].

Additional examinations, aimed at excluding lesions of the central nervous system, include brain imaging methods (CT or MRI examination), neurological examination (EEG, evoked potentials), psychological and neuropsychological examination [Ministarstvo zdravlja Republike Srbije, 2011].

When it comes to depressive episodes of mild to moderate intensity, according to ICD-10, it is possible to record the presence or absence of somatic symptoms. When it comes to depression with somatic complaints, in addition to the presence of a mild or moderately severe depressive episode, 4 to 8 of the following items are required (Somatic symptoms of depression, simplified according to ICD-10) [WHO, 1992]:

1. Anhedonia,

2. Lack of response to events/activities that normally provoke an emotional response,

3. Early morning awakening,

4. Morning worsening of depression,

5. Psychomotor retardation/agitation,

6. Significant loss of appetite,

7. Weight loss,

8. Loss of libido.

In summary, the diagnostic criteria for depressive disorder are presented in Table 5.

Table 5. Diagnosis of depressive disorder according to ICD-10

Symptoms of a depressive episode	Depressive episodes by severity and quality
Typical symptoms 1. Depressed mood 2. Loss of interest and pleasure 3. Decreased energy, increased fatigue, decreased activity	Mild depressive episode (2 typical + 2 other symptoms) Moderately severe depressive episode (2 typical + 3 or 4 other symptoms) Major depressive episode without psychotic symptoms (3 typical + 4 or more other symptoms) Major depressive episode with psychotic symptoms* (3 typical + 4 or more of the others + psychotic symptoms) *Psychotic symptoms (delusions: misery, guilt, hypochondriacal, nihilistic and others; hallucinations; depressive stupor)
	Depressive episode with somatic symptoms
Other common symptoms (other symptoms)	Somatic symptoms*

a) impaired concentration and attention	> loss of interest or pleasure in activities that normally bring pleasure
b) decreased self-confidence and self-esteem	> lack of emotional response to pleasant events and surroundings
c) feelings of guilt and worthlessness (even in mild depression)	> waking up two or more hours earlier than usual
d) gloomy and pessimistic view of the future	> depression worse in the morning
e) thoughts of self-harm or suicide	> clear psychomotor retardation or agitation
f) disturbed sleep	> marked loss of appetite
g) decreased appetite	> weight loss (5% or more in the last month)
Duration of symptoms for at least two weeks	> marked loss of libido *at least 4 of the listed symptoms are present for mild and moderate depressive episodes, specifically mark; implied for severe depressive episode
	Depressive episode with psychotic symptoms
	Psychotic symptoms* > delusions or hallucinations, most often with guilt, depressive, hypochondriac or nihilistic content, ideas of relationships or ideas of persecution > depressed stupor > mood-congruent psychotic symptoms (e.g., delusions of guilt, worthlessness, somatic illness, or impending doom; mocking or judgmental hallucinations) > mood-incongruent psychotic symptoms (e.g., delusions of persecution and relationships, hallucinations without affective content)

	*Psychotic symptoms may only occur in severe depressive episodes
Duration of symptoms for at least two weeks	

Source: [Ministarstvo zdravlja Republike Srbije, 2011, p. 18]

When delusions, hallucinations, or stupor are present, a diagnosis of psychotic depression is made, and psychotic symptoms may or may not be consistent with mood.

Dysthymia, in which the criteria for a depressive episode are not met, lasts at least two years, and is classified as a persistent mood disorder. The diagnostic criteria for dysthymia, also called chronic depression, are presented in Table 6.

Table 6. Diagnostic criteria for dysthymia (according to ICD-10)

A. A period of at least two years of constant or consistently recurrent depressed mood. Interspersed periods of normal mood rarely lasting more than a few weeks. No episodes of hypomania
B. No episodes of depression (or very few) in that two-year period are severe or long-lasting enough to meet the diagnostic criteria for recurrent, mild depressive disorder.
C. During at least some episodes of depression, at least three of the following symptoms must be present: 1. decreased energy or activity 2. insomnia 3. loss of self-confidence or feelings of inadequacy 4. difficulty concentrating 5. frequent crying 6. loss of interest or pleasure in sex and other pleasurable activities 7. feelings of hopelessness or despair 8. feelings of inability to cope with the routine responsibilities of daily life 9. pessimism about the future or excessive thinking about the past 10. social withdrawal 11. decreased talkativeness

Note: if necessary, the time of onset can be designated as early (in the late teens or twenties) or late (usually between the ages of 30 and 50, followed by a single affective episode).

Source: [Ministarstvo zdravlja Republike Srbije, 2011, p. 19]

Diagnosing depression is crucial not only for its treatment but also for the prevention of suicide. According to previous research, about two-thirds of suicides are committed by people suffering from depression. Individuals suffering from depression, especially those with severe depression, are 4 to 20 times more likely to commit suicide than the general population [Ministarstvo zdravlja Republike Srbije, 2011].

2.5. Hamilton Depression Rating Scale

Controlled clinical studies objectify clinical assessment using scales as basic instruments. Scales allow the presence/absence of symptoms, their intensity, to assess significant clinical parameters for certain entities and to express all this in figures and numbers, without changing the clinical assessment. Scales are quantified and are suitable for statistical processing. Based on this, scales for assessing depressive disorders are widely used and useful in the clinical work of psychiatrists.

Among the scales for assessing depression, the Hamilton Depression Scale (HAM) has a significant place. Hamilton Depression Rating Scale (HAM-D) [Hamilton, 1986] is highly reliable and valid and is one of the most widely used scales in research. This scale is one of the best known and most frequently used for assessing depression (e.g. [Wang et al., 2022; Akpinar et al., 2022; Shahid et al., 2011]). It consists of twenty-one (21) questions with the possibility of ranking the answers on a four-point scale from 0 to 3, where higher values on the scale indicate the presence of more intense depressive symptoms. The total score is calculated by simply adding all the answers, and the total score values range from 0 to 63. The scale is widely used in everyday work with depressed patients and in research. It can be used with psychiatric, non-psychiatric patients and healthy populations.

[1] *Lacasse Y, Rousseau L, Maltais F. Prevalence of depressive symptoms and depression in patients with severe oxygen-dependent chronic obstructive pulmonary disease. Journal of Cardiopulmonary Rehabilitation and Prevention. 2001 Mar 1;21(2):80-6.*
[2] *Wong TS, Xiang YT, Tsoh J, Ungvari GS, Ko FW, Hui DS, Chiu HF. Depressive disorders in older patients with chronic obstructive pulmonary disease (COPD) in Hong Kong: a controlled study. Aging & mental health. 2014 Jul 4;18(5):588-92.*
[3] *Yao HM, Xiao RS, Cao PL, Wang XL, Zuo W, Zhang W. Risk factors for depression in patients with chronic obstructive pulmonary disease. World Journal of Psychiatry. 2020 Apr 4;10(4):59.*
[4] *Kim KU, Park HK, Jung HY, Ahn JJ, Moon E, Kim YS, Lee MK, Lee H. Association of depression with disease severity in patients with chronic obstructive pulmonary disease. Lung. 2014 Apr;192:243-9.*
[5] *Lou P, Zhu Y, Chen P, Zhang P, Yu J, Wang Y, Chen N, Zhang L, Wu H, Zhao J. Interaction of depressive and anxiety symptoms on the mortality of patients with COPD: a preliminary study. COPD: Journal of Chronic Obstructive Pulmonary Disease. 2014 Aug 1;11(4):444-50.*
[6] *Maurer J, Rebbapragada V, Borson S, Goldstein R, Kunik ME, Yohannes AM, Hanania NA. Anxiety and depression in COPD: current understanding, unanswered questions, and research needs. Chest. 2008 Oct 1;134(4):43S-56S.*
[7] *Katon W, Ciechanowski P. Impact of major depression on chronic medical illness. Journal of psychosomatic research. 2002 Oct 1;53(4):859-63.*
[8] *Fritzsche A, Clamor A, von Leupoldt A. Effects of medical and psychological treatment of depression in patients with COPD–a review. Respiratory medicine. 2011 Oct 1;105(10):1422-33.*
[9] *Billings AG, Moos RH. Comparisons of children of depressed and nondepressed parents: A social-environmental perspective. Journal of Abnormal Child Psychology. 1983 Dec;11:463-85.*
[10] *Brown J, Cohen P, Johnson JG, Smailes EM. Childhood abuse and neglect: specificity of effects on adolescent and young adult depression and suicidality. Journal of the American Academy of Child & Adolescent Psychiatry. 1999 Dec 1;38(12):1490-6.*
[11] *Maharaj S, Lees T, Lal S. Prevalence and risk factors of depression, anxiety, and stress in a cohort of Australian nurses. International journal of environmental research and public health. 2019 Jan;16(1):61.*
[12] *Solé B, Verdolini N, Amoretti S, Montejo L, Rosa AR, Hogg B, Garcia-Rizo C, Mezquida G, Bernardo M, Martinez-Aran A, Vieta E. Effects of the COVID-19 pandemic and lockdown in Spain: comparison between community controls and patients with a psychiatric disorder. Preliminary results from the BRIS-MHC STUDY. Journal of affective disorders. 2021*

Feb 15;281:13-23.

[13]*LaGrant B, Marquis BO, Berg AT, Grinspan ZM. Depression and anxiety in children with epilepsy and other chronic health conditions: national estimates of prevalence and risk factors. Epilepsy & Behavior. 2020 Feb 1;103:106828.*

[14]*Gray C, Ambady L, Chao S, Smith W, Yoon J. Virtual Management of Chronic Conditions During the COVID-19 Pandemic: Insights From Primary Care Providers and Clinical Pharmacists. Military Medicine. 2023 Jul 1;188(7-8):e2615-20.*

[15]*Balcells E, Gea J, Ferrer J, Serra I, Orozco-Levi M, de Batlle J, Rodriguez E, Benet M, Donaire-González D, Antó JM, Garcia-Aymerich J. Factors affecting the relationship between psychological status and quality of life in COPD patients. Health and quality of life outcomes. 2010 Dec;8:1-9.*

[16]*Sundh J, Ställberg B, Lisspers K, Montgomery SM, Janson C. Co-morbidity, body mass index and quality of life in COPD using the Clinical COPD Questionnaire. COPD: Journal of Chronic Obstructive Pulmonary Disease. 2011 May 27;8(3):173-81.*

[17]*Pedrozo-Pupo JC, Campo-Arias A, Ceballos-Ospino GA. Quality of life and depression in COPD patients in the Colombian Caribbean. The Clinical Respiratory Journal. 2021 Sep;15(9):944-8.*

[18]*Fan VS, Ramsey SD, Giardino ND, Make BJ, Emery CF, Diaz PT, Benditt JO, Mosenifar Z, McKenna R, Curtis JL, Fishman AP. Sex, depression, and risk of hospitalization and mortality in chronic obstructive pulmonary disease. Archives of internal medicine. 2007 Nov 26;167(21):2345-53.*

[19]*Cafarella PA, Effing TW, USMANI ZA, Frith PA. Treatments for anxiety and depression in patients with chronic obstructive pulmonary disease: a literature review. Respirology. 2012 May;17(4):627-38.*

[20]*Yohannes AM, Hann M, Sibbald B. The management of depressive symptoms in patients with COPD: a postal survey of general practitioners. Primary health care research & development. 2011 Jul;12(3):237-44.*

[21]*Lin P, Campbell DG, Chaney EF, Liu CF, Heagerty P, Felker BL, Hedrick SC. The influence of patient preference on depression treatment in primary care. Annals of Behavioral Medicine. 2005 Oct 1;30(2):164-73.*

[22]*Yohannes AM, Jin JW, Kunik ME. Benefit–risk assessment of psychotropic drugs in older patients with chronic obstructive pulmonary disease. Drugs & Aging. 2022 May;39(5):323-32.*

[23]*Yohannes AM, Leroi I. Pharmacological therapy and anxiolytics in patients with respiratory diseases. Depression and anxiety in patients with chronic respiratory diseases. 2017:167-82*

[24]*Tselebis A, Pachi A, Ilias I, Kosmas E, Bratis D, Moussas G, Tzanakis N. Strategies to improve anxiety and depression in patients with COPD: a*

mental health perspective. Neuropsychiatric disease and treatment. 2016 Feb 9:297-328.

[25]*Zuo M, Huang Y, Ma W, Xue Z, Zhang J, Gong Y, Che L. Expert recommendations for tracheal intubation in critically ill patients with noval coronavirus disease 2019. Chinese Medical Sciences Journal. 2020 Jun 1;35(2):105-9.*

[26]*Chanques G, Constantin JM, Devlin JW, Ely EW, Fraser GL, Gélinas C, Girard TD, Guérin C, Jabaudon M, Jaber S, Mehta S. Analgesia and sedation in patients with ARDS. Intensive care medicine. 2020 Dec;46:2342-56.*

[27]*Keller MB, McCullough JP, Klein DN, Arnow B, Dunner DL, Gelenberg AJ, Markowitz JC, Nemeroff CB, Russell JM, Thase ME, Trivedi MH. A comparison of nefazodone, the cognitive behavioral-analysis system of psychotherapy, and their combination for the treatment of chronic depression. New England journal of medicine. 2000 May 18;342(20):1462-70.*

[28]*von Wietersheim J, Kessler H. Psychotherapy with chronic inflammatory bowel disease patients: a review. Inflammatory bowel diseases. 2006 Dec 1;12(12):1175-84.*

[29]*Hamilton J, Guthrie E, Creed F, Thompson D, Tomenson B, Bennett R, Moriarty K, Stephens W, Liston R. A randomized controlled trial of psychotherapy in patients with chronic functional dyspepsia. Gastroenterology. 2000 Sep 1;119(3):661-9.*

[30]*Nemeroff CB, Heim CM, Thase ME, Klein DN, Rush AJ, Schatzberg AF, Ninan PT, McCullough Jr JP, Weiss PM, Dunner DL, Rothbaum BO. Differential responses to psychotherapy versus pharmacotherapy in patients with chronic forms of major depression and childhood trauma. Proceedings of the National Academy of Sciences. 2003 Nov 25;100(24):14293-6.*

[31]*Schramm E, Kriston L, Elsaesser M, Fangmeier T, Meister R, Bausch P, Zobel I, Bailer J, Wambach K, Backenstrass M, Klein JP. Two-year follow-up after treatment with the cognitive behavioral analysis system of psychotherapy versus supportive psychotherapy for early-onset chronic depression. Psychotherapy and psychosomatics. 2019;88(3):154-64.*

[32]*Urtasun M, Daray FM, Teti GL, Coppolillo F, Herlax G, Saba G, Rubinstein A, Araya R, Irazola V. Validation and calibration of the patient health questionnaire (PHQ-9) in Argentina. BMC psychiatry. 2019 Dec;19(1):1-0.*

[33]*Ivana Jelić, Goran Mihajlović, Jovanka Kos, Učestalost simptoma*

depresije i depresivne epizode u primarnoj zdravstvenoj zaštiti, Engrami 2013; 35(1):5-11.
[34]*Story DA, Tait AR. Survey research. Anesthesiology. 2019 Feb;130(2):192-202.*
[35]*Morin Amy LCSW. 2021. Screening for Depression: How Depression Tests Work. May 28, 2021. https://www.verywellmind.com/depression-tests-mood-disorder-4174922*
[36]*APA. Depression Assessment Instruments. These instruments are relevant to the treatment of depression. 2023. https://www.apa.org/depression-guideline/assessment*
[37]*Ayalon L, Goldfracht M, Bech P. 'Do you think you suffer from depression?'Reevaluating the use of a single item question for the screening of depression in older primary care patients. International Journal of Geriatric Psychiatry: A journal of the psychiatry of late life and allied sciences. 2010 May;25(5):497-502.*
[38]*Manea L, Gilbody S, McMillan D. Optimal cut-off score for diagnosing depression with the Patient Health Questionnaire (PHQ-9): a meta-analysis. Cmaj. 2012 Feb 21;184(3):E191-6.*
[39]*Ministarstvo zdravlja Republike Srbije. 2011. Национални водич добре клиничке праксе. Депресија. https://www.zdravlje.gov.rs/view_file.php?file_id=675&cache=sr;*
[40]*Jelić I, Mihajlović G, Mihajlović F, Minić N, Ratinac M, Pantović-Stefanović M. COPD and Depression Analysis in Regard to Obstructive Pulmonary Levels. In Healthcare 2023 Apr 19 (Vol. 11, No. 8, p. 1175). MDPI.*
[41]*Peterson JB. Maps of meaning: The architecture of belief. Routledge; 2002 Sep 11.*
[42]*Ministarstvo zdravlja i socijalne zaštite Republike Srpske. Klinički vodič - Duševni poremećaji i poremećaji ponašanja. 2008. https://www.vladars.net/sr-SP-Cyrl/Vlada/Ministarstva/MZSZ/Documents/depresija_distimija.pdf*
[43]*Bromet E, Andrade LH, Hwang I, Sampson NA, Alonso J, De Girolamo G, De Graaf R, Demyttenaere K, Hu C, Iwata N, Karam AN. Cross-national epidemiology of DSM-IV major depressive episode. BMC medicine. 2011 Dec;9(1):1-6.*
[44]*Waraich P, Goldner EM, Somers JM, Hsu L. Prevalence and incidence studies of mood disorders: a systematic review of the literature. The Canadian Journal of Psychiatry. 2004 Feb;49(2):124-38.*
[45]*Daly M. Prevalence of depression among adolescents in the US from 2009 to 2019: analysis of trends by sex, race/ethnicity, and income. Journal of*

Adolescent Health. 2022 Mar 1;70(3):496-9.
[46]*WHO. World Health Organization. 2021. World health statistics 2021: monitoring health for the SDGs, sustainable development goals. https://www.who.int/publications/i/item/9789240027053*
[47]*WHO. World Health Organization. 2022. World health statistics 2022: monitoring health for the SDGs, sustainable development goals. https://www.who.int/publications/i/item/9789240051157*
[48]*Lépine JP, Briley M. The increasing burden of depression. Neuropsychiatric disease and treatment. 2011 May 31;7(sup1):3-7.*
[49]*Baxter AJ, Scott KM, Ferrari AJ, Norman RE, Vos T, Whiteford HA. Challenging the myth of an "epidemic" of common mental disorders: trends in the global prevalence of anxiety and depression between 1990 and 2010. Depression and anxiety. 2014 Jun;31(6):506-16.*
[50]*Greenberg PE, Fournier AA, Sisitsky T, Pike CT, Kessler RC. The economic burden of adults with major depressive disorder in the United States (2005 and 2010). The Journal of clinical psychiatry. 2015 Feb 25;76(2):5356.*
[51]*Peterson JB. Maps of meaning: The architecture of belief. Routledge; 2002 Sep 11.*
[52]*Ministarstvo zdravlja i socijalne zaštite Republike Srpske. Klinički vodič - Duševni poremećaji i poremećaji ponašanja. 2008. https://www.vladars.net/sr-SP-Cyrl/Vlada/Ministarstva/MZSZ/Documents/depresija_distimija.pdf*
[53]*Bromet E, Andrade LH, Hwang I, Sampson NA, Alonso J, De Girolamo G, De Graaf R, Demyttenaere K, Hu C, Iwata N, Karam AN. Cross-national epidemiology of DSM-IV major depressive episode. BMC medicine. 2011 Dec;9(1):1-6.*
[54]*Waraich P, Goldner EM, Somers JM, Hsu L. Prevalence and incidence studies of mood disorders: a systematic review of the literature. The Canadian Journal of Psychiatry. 2004 Feb;49(2):124-38.*
[55]*Daly M. Prevalence of depression among adolescents in the US from 2009 to 2019: analysis of trends by sex, race/ethnicity, and income. Journal of Adolescent Health. 2022 Mar 1;70(3):496-9.*
[56]*WHO. World Health Organization. 2021. World health statistics 2021: monitoring health for the SDGs, sustainable development goals. https://www.who.int/publications/i/item/9789240027053*
[57]*WHO. World Health Organization. 2022. World health statistics 2022: monitoring health for the SDGs, sustainable development goals. https://www.who.int/publications/i/item/9789240051157*
[58]*Lépine JP, Briley M. The increasing burden of depression. Neuropsychiatric disease and treatment. 2011 May 31;7(sup1):3-7.*
Baxter AJ, Scott KM, Ferrari AJ, Norman RE, Vos T, Whiteford HA.

Challenging the myth of an "epidemic" of common mental disorders: trends in the global prevalence of anxiety and depression between 1990 and 2010. Depression and anxiety. 2014 Jun;31(6):506-16.

[59]*Greenberg PE, Fournier AA, Sisitsky T, Pike CT, Kessler RC. The economic burden of adults with major depressive disorder in the United States (2005 and 2010). The Journal of clinical psychiatry. 2015 Feb 25;76(2):5356.*

[60]*O'Connor EA, Whitlock EP, Gaynes B, Beil TL. Screening for depression in adults and older adults in primary care: an updated systematic review. https://www.ncbi.nlm.nih.gov/books/NBK36410/*

[61]*Williams LJ, Pasco JA, Jackson H, Kiropoulos L, Stuart AL, Jacka FN, Berk M. Depression as a risk factor for fracture in women: a 10 year longitudinal study. Journal of affective disorders. 2016 Mar 1;192:34-40.*

[62]*Siniscalchi KA, Broome ME, Fish J, Ventimiglia J, Thompson J, Roy P, Pipes R, Trivedi M. Depression screening and measurement-based care in primary care. Journal of primary care & community health. 2020 Nov;11:2150132720931261. https://www.ncbi.nlm.nih.gov/pmc/articles/PMC7673056/*

[63]*NCHC. National Center for Health Statistics. 2023. Depression. Morbidity. https://www.cdc.gov/nchs/data/nhis/earlyrelease/EarlyRelease202009-508.pdf.*

[64]*NCHC. National Center for Health Statistics. 2023. National Ambulatory Medical Care Survey: 2019 National Summary Tables. https://www.cdc.gov/nchs/data/ahcd/namcs_summary/2019-namcs-web-tables-508.pdf.*

[65]*NCHC. National Center for Health Statistics. 2023. Antidepressant Use Among Adults: United States, 2015-2018. https://www.cdc.gov/nchs/products/databriefs/db377.htm.*

[66]*NCHC. National Center for Health Statistics. 2023. Depression. https://www.cdc.gov/nchs/fastats/depression.htm*

[67]*Gustavson K, Knudsen AK, Nesvåg R, Knudsen GP, Vollset SE, Reichborn-Kjennerud T. Prevalence and stability of mental disorders among young adults: findings from a longitudinal study. BMC psychiatry. 2018 Dec;18:1-5.*

[68]*Hansen T, Slagsvold B. The East–West divide in late-life depression in Europe: results from the Generations and Gender Survey. Scandinavian psychologist. 2017 Mar 8;4.*

[69]*Van Winkle Z, Ferragina E, Recchi E. The unexpected decline in feelings of depression among adults ages 50 and older in 11 European countries amid the COVID-19 pandemic. Socius. 2021 Aug;7:23780231211032741.*

[70]*Eurostat. Reporting cronic depression (10. september 2021). 2021. https://ec.europa.eu/eurostat/web/products-eurostat-news/-/edn-20210910-1*

[71]*ECDC. European Centre for Disease Prevention and Control. 2023.*

https://www.ecdc.europa.eu/en
[72]*Van de Velde S, Bracke P, Levecque K. Gender differences in depression in 23 European countries. Cross-national variation in the gender gap in depression. Social science & medicine. 2010 Jul 1;71(2):305-13.*
[73]*Ibrahim AK, Kelly SJ, Adams CE, Glazebrook C. A systematic review of studies of depression prevalence in university students. Journal of psychiatric research. 2013 Mar 1;47(3):391-400.*
[74]*Arias-de la Torre J, Vilagut G, Ronaldson A, Serrano-Blanco A, Martín V, Peters M, Valderas JM, Dregan A, Alonso J. Prevalence and variability of current depressive disorder in 27 European countries: a population-based study. The Lancet Public Health. 2021 Oct 1;6(10):e729-38.*
[75]*Pravno informacioni sistem Repblike Srbije. Program o zaštiti mentalnog zdravlja u Republici Srbiji za period 2019–2026. godine. „Službeni glasnik RS", broj 84 od 29. novembra 2019. 2019. https://www.pravno-informacionisistem.rs/SlGlasnikPortal/eli/rep/sgrs/vlada/drugiakt/2019/84/1*
.
[76]*Martinović I. Pet odsto stanovništva Srbije u depresiji. 12. februar 2019. 2019. https://www.slobodnaevropa.org/a/pet-odsto-stanovnistva-srbije-u-depresiji/29764316.html*
[77]*WHO. Fact sheet on Sustainable Development Goals (SDGs): health targets. Mental health. 2018.*
[78]*WHO. Depression and other common mental disorders: global health estimates. World Health Organization. Geneva. 2017. https://apps.who.int/iris/handle/10665/254610*
[79]*Jaffe DH, Rive B, Denee TR. The humanistic and economic burden of treatment-resistant depression in Europe: a cross-sectional study. BMC psychiatry. 2019 Dec;19:1-1.*
[80]*Batut. Institut za javno zdravlje Srbije „Dr Milan Jovanović Batut", Zdravstveno statistički godišnjak. Studija „Istraživanje zdravlja stanovništva Srbije 2019. godine"; 2019. https://www.batut.org.rs/download/publikacije/ZdravljeStanovnistva2019.pdf*
[81]*Batut. Institut za javno zdravlje Srbije „Dr Milan Jovanović Batut", Zdravstveno statistički godišnjak. 2011.*
[82]*Greenberg PE, Fournier AA, Sisitsky T, Simes M, Berman R, Koenigsberg SH, Kessler RC. The economic burden of adults with major depressive disorder in the United States (2010 and 2018). Pharmacoeconomics. 2021 Jun;39(6):653-65. https://pubmed.ncbi.nlm.nih.gov/33950419/*
[83]*APA. The Economic Cost of Depression is Increasing; Direct Costs are Only a Small Part. May 27, 2021. https://www.psychiatry.org/News-room/APA-Blogs/The-Economic-Cost-of-Depression-is-Increasing*

[84]*Keshavarz K, Hedayati A, Rezaei M, Goudarzi Z, Moghimi E, Rezaee M, Lotfi F. Economic burden of major depressive disorder: a case study in Southern Iran. BMC psychiatry. 2022 Aug 30;22(1):577.*
[85]*Johnston KM, Powell LC, Anderson IM, Szabo S, Cline S. The burden of treatment-resistant depression: a systematic review of the economic and quality of life literature. Journal of affective disorders. 2019 Jan 1;242:195-210.*
[86]*Goldenberg DL. Diagnosis and differential diagnosis of fibromyalgia. The American journal of medicine. 2009 Dec 1;122(12):S14-21.*
[87]*Kimmel PL, Weihs K, Peterson RA. Survival in hemodialysis patients: the role of depression. Journal of the American Society of Nephrology. 1993 Jul 1;4(1):12-27.*
[88]*Gruenberg AM, Goldstein RD, Pincus HA. Classification of depression: Research and diagnostic criteria: DSM-IV and ICD-10. Biology of depression: From novel insights to therapeutic strategies. 2005 Jan 26:1-2.*
[89]*Löwe B, Gräfe K, Zipfel S, Witte S, Loerch B, Herzog W. Diagnosing ICD-10 depressive episodes: superior criterion validity of the Patient Health Questionnaire. Psychotherapy and psychosomatics. 2004;73(6):386-90.*
[90]*WHO. The ICD-10 classification of mental and behavioural disorders: clinical descriptions and diagnostic guidelines. World Health Organization; 1992.*
[91]*Rizzo R, Piccinelli M, Mazzi MA, Bellantuono C, Tansella M. The Personal Health Questionnaire: a new screening instrument for detection of ICD-10 depressive disorders in primary care. Psychological Medicine. 2000 Jul;30(4):831-40.*

PART THREE

Quality of Life – COPD and Depression

3. Quality of Life – Chronic Obstructive Pulmonary Disease and Depression

Quality of life is studied in various fields and depends on people's perceptions [Cummnins RA, 2000; An et al., 2021]. Research on people's quality of life began to develop after World War II, initially in the USA where the financial situation of an individual was one of the main components of life satisfaction [Cummnins RA, 2000; Schalock R, 2000; Wojewódzka-Wiewiórska A et al., 2019; Aria M et al., 2020]. On the other hand, during the 1960s, research indicated that the subjective feeling of satisfaction and happiness are important for quality of life [Wojewódzka-Wiewiórska A et al., 2019; Aria M et al., 2020; Allison PJ et al., 1997]. Therefore, it can be argued that quality of life is the sum of the subjective feeling of satisfaction with life and other circumstances such as living conditions, financial situation, personal values, personal progress and the like [Borthwick-Duffy SA, 2000; O'Boyle C, 1994; Jelić I et al., 2021; Sirgy MJ, 2021; Hall A, 2020].

Quality of life is, therefore, the sum of a series of facts of subjective and objective aspects of an individual's life [Sirgy MJ, 2021; Zapf W et al., 1984; Felce D et al., 1995; Mount BM et al., 1995; Veenhoven R, 2000].

3.1. The Definition of the Quality of Life

When it comes to defining the quality of life in relation to health, there are many definitions that have emerged because of the understanding that health is one of the most important conditions for a good quality of life. The WHO indicates that it is not only the duration of life that is important, but also the quality of life. Regarding the connection between quality of life and health, a group of experts from the WHO provides a definition of life that is considered the most comprehensive:

> Quality of life is defined as the perception of individuals about their own position in life in the context of the culture and value system in which they live, as well as according to their goals, expectations, standards and interests [WHO, 1998].

In addition, the WHO defines health not only as the absence of disease but as complete physical, mental and social well-being. Also, the WHO defines 6 dimensions that make up quality of life:

1. physical domain,
2. psychological domain,
3. level of independence,
4. social relationships,
5. environment and
6. spirituality (religion, personal beliefs).

Based on this, it can be argued that quality of life is a cognitive process that identifies mental health, perceived health, physical function and social function [WHO, 1998].

Methods of examining quality of life are different. For this type of examination, some of the questionnaires for assessing quality of life are used, because questionnaires are precisely the instruments for measuring the quality of life [Dugalić S, 2016; Ristić Ž, 2016; Krabbe PF, 2008]. Namely, at the end of the 19th century, the first results of research and measurement scales conducted in the field of psychiatry were described, namely by Thurstone [Thurstone LL, 1927] and Likert [Likert R, 1932]. Since then, the concept of Health-Related Quality of Life (HRQoL) has emerged because of the assertion that health is the most important condition for a good quality of life.

In routine practice, an approach that defines the quality of life of a patient through the patient's assessment in four areas is increasingly used. It includes:

- physical and professional ability,
- psychological state,
- social activities and
- somatic complaints.

In our country, several scientific meetings have been organized by the Serbian Academy of Sciences and Arts (SANU) on the definition and evaluation of the quality of life of patients with inflammatory diseases. The importance of this topic is also evidenced by the fact that the professional community is actively indicating that, for the health status of patients, it is necessary to conduct measurements of quality of life in relation to health, in addition to the usual clinical measurements [Radovanović N et al., 2008; Zdravković M et al., 2010;

Terzić Z et al., 2005; Jocić Stojanović J et al., 2015; Gvozdenović B et al., 2007]. In this case, the patient is his or her own control, and the comparison is made in relation to the patient's expected abilities.

It is important to obtain a complete health status of the patients, because often patients with the same somatic complaints do not have the same subjective complaints that the disease leads to, and which are important for the patients in their daily functioning [Ursin H, 1997; North CS et al., 2007; Eriksen HR et al., 2004]. For these reasons, it is necessary to conduct a health-related quality of life measurement in addition to the usual clinical measurements. The measurement of the quality of life should not focus exclusively on the diseased organ or organ system, but should also include the physical, social and emotional disorders that the patients experience because of the primary disease and that the patients face.

Previous research has shown that a proper assessment of quality of life achieves an easier choice of priorities in planning therapeutic procedures, faster and better communication between doctors and patients, as well as a simple observation of potential problems of the patients. It is also the most accurate way to find out how realistic the patients' expectations of the treatment are, measures of monitoring changes during treatment, the quality of care provided to patients, and the outcome of the overall treatment [Kulić L et al., 2019].

In recent years, many questionnaires have been developed as instruments for measuring the quality of life [Garratt A et al., 2002; Theofilou P, 2013; Morris J et al., 1997; Mooney A, 2006; Acquadro C et al., 2008; Swaine-Verdier A et al., 2004; Haraldstad K et al., 2019]. According to their structure, they are divided into general (generic) and specific (disease-specific questionnaires). Which instrument will be used during the study program is determined by the physician according to the clinical problem and the measurement characteristics of the instrument.

3.2. General (generic) Questionnaires for Assessing the Quality of Life in Patients with Chronic Obstructive Pulmonary Disease and Depression

Of great importance in assessing the quality of life of patients with COPD and depression is the choice of the type of questionnaire that will be used in the study. It is necessary that the questionnaire has a certain specificity of the disease and objectively measures the quality of life of the patient.

Various questionnaires have been used in previous studies:

• Short-form 36 questionnaire (SF-36),

• Nottingham Health Profile (NHP) questionnaire,

• Psychological General Wellbeing Index (PGWI),

• Physical Activity Score (PAS),

• Minnesota Living with Heart Failure Questionnaire,

• Quality of Life Enjoyment and Satisfaction Questionnaire (Q-LES-Q).

One of the most reliable questionnaires is the Q-LES-Q-SF (Quality of Life and Life Satisfaction Questionnaire), which very realistically reflects the quality of life and has an excellent correlation with both the physical and mental capabilities of the patient (see [Lee YT et al., 2014; Stevanovic D et al., 2011].

3.3. Q-LES-Q – Questionnaire for Measuring Quality of Life and Life Satisfaction

The Q-LES-Q is a questionnaire for measuring general quality of life. The questionnaire is a psychometrically valid, effective way of measuring and allows for comparison of quality of life in different diseases and populations. It was developed in the USA in the late 1980s as part of the Medical Outcomes Study (MOS), a longitudinal study of self-assessment of the health status of patients with various chronic conditions [Revicki DA et al., 2014; Michalak EE et al., 2007]. The questionnaire on the quality of life and satisfaction contains dimensions such as physical health, mental state, work/job, home activities, leisure activities and social relationships [Riendeau RP et al., 2018; Endicott J et al., 1993; WHO, 1996].

3.4. Measuring the Quality of Life

Emotional changes, such as depression, in patients with COPD are mainly due to the high severity of the disease. This degree of disease is associated with physical disability, but also with reduced quality of life and increased use of health services. In addition, the presence of depression worsens clinical symptoms in patients in both the short and long term [Norwood RJ, 2007; Martinez RC et al., 2016; Jelić et al., 2023; Stage KB et al., 2006]. Due to the complexity of COPD and its multiple components, in addition to the chronicity with which it occurs, treatment is necessary for recovery but also for improving the quality of life. Primarily, treatment is based on the eradication of smoking as the main cause of the disease, which is considered the most effective measure to prevent the progression of this disease as well as to eradicate it [Tønnesen P, 2013; Bai JW et al., 2017]. Associated with depression, patients with COPD are also subject to drug therapy based mainly on antidepressants [Fritzsche A et al., 2011; Yohannes AM et al., 2014; Deb A et al., 2017].

There are several studies that have examined the quality of life of patients with chronic lung inflammation before and after drug treatment (e.g. antidepressants) ([Siraj RA et al., 2002]. As COPD is a very common disease of modern times, examining the quality of life in these patients is important not only for patients, but also for physicians. It is especially important for health care funding and planning [Buttery SC et al., 2021].

---

[1]*Cummnins RA. Objective and subjective quality of life: an interactive model. Soc Indic Res. 2000; 52: 55-72.*

[2]*An J, Zhou H, Yang T, Duan C, Bao C, Wan C, Shen Y, Wen F. Relationship of psychological factors with daily activities and quality of life in patients with chronic obstructive pulmonary disease in a Chinese rural population. Annals of palliative medicine. 2021 Feb 1;10(2):1675-84.*

[3]*Schalock R. Three decades of quality of life. Focus Autism Other Dev Disabl. 2000; 15(2):116-27.*

[4]*Wojewódzka-Wiewiórska A, Kłoczko-Gajewska A, Sulewski P. Between the social and economic dimensions of sustainability in rural areas—in search of farmers' quality of life. Sustainability. 2019 Dec 23;12(1):148.*

[5]*Aria M, Misuraca M, Spano M. Mapping the evolution of social research and data science on 30 years of social indicators research. Social indicators research. 2020 Jun;149:803-31.*

[6]*Allison PJ, Locker D, Feine JS. Quality of life: a dynamic construct. Soc Sci Med. 1997; 45(2): 221-30.*

[7]*Borthwick-Duffy SA. Quality of life and quality of care in mental retardation. Mental retardation in the year 2000. Berlin: Ed. L. Rowitz; 1992. p. 52-66.*

[8]*O'Boyle C. The Schedule for the evaluation of individual Quality of life (SEI-QOL). Int J Ment Health. 1994; 23(3): 3-23.*

[9]*Ivana Jelić, Marko Folic, Filip Mihajlović, Slobodan Janković, Goran Mihajlović, The effects of antidepressant therapy on health-related quality of life in patients with a chronic obstructive pulmonary disease and depressive*

symptoms, Serbian Journal of experimental and Clinical Research 2021;doi: 10.2478/sjecr-2021-0068.

[10]*Sirgy MJ. The psychology of quality of life: Wellbeing and positive mental health. Social Indicators Research Series. Springer International Publishing, Cham. https://doi. org/10.1007/978-3-030-71888-6. 2021.*

Hall A. Quality of life and value assessment in health care. Health Care Analysis. 2020 Mar;28(1):45-61.

[11]*Zapf W, Glatzer W. German Social Report: Living Conditions and Subjective Well-Being. Soc Indic Res. 1984; 19: 1-171.*

[12]*Felce D, Perry J. Quality of life: its definition and measurement. Res Dev Disabil.1995; 16(1): 51-74.*

[13]*Mount BM, Cohen SR. Quality of life in the face of life-threatening illnes: What should we be measuring? Current Oncology 1995; 2: 121-25.*

Veenhoven R. The four Qualities of life Ordering concepts and measures of the good life. J Happiness Stud. 2000; 1(1): 1-39.

[14]*WHO. The World Health Organization Quality of Life Assessment –WHO-QoL, 1998.*

[15]*Dugalić S. Značaj sporta i ponašanja sportista za formiranje stavova ljudi. SPORT-Nauka i Praksa, 5. 2016;22.*

[16]*Ristić Ž. Objedinjavanje kvantitativnih i kvalitativnih istraživanja. Beograd: Evropski centar za mir i razvoj – Univerzitet za mir Ujedinjenih nacija. 2016.*

[17]*Krabbe PF. Thurstone scaling as a measurement method to quantify subjective health outcomes. Medical care. 2008 Apr 1:357-65.*

Thurstone LL. A law of comparative judgments. Psychol Rev. 1927;34: 273–286.

[18]*Likert R. A technique for the measurement of attitudes. Archives of psychology. 1932.*

[19]*Radovanović N, Jakovljević Đ, Kanjuh V. Quality of life after open heart surgery: a ten year follow-up research study. U: Kanjuh V, Radovanović N, eds. Atherothrombotic coronary heart disease: morphological-clinical correlations. Belgrade: Serbian Academy of Sciences and Arts; 2008.*

[20]*Zdravković M, Krotin M, Deljanin-Ilić M, Zdravković D. Merenje kvaliteta života bolesnika sa kardiovaskularnim oboljenjima. Medicinski pregled. 2010;9:10.*

[21]*Terzić Z, Bjegović V, Marinković J, Draganić G, Ljubić B, Seferović J. Merenje kvaliteta života bolesnika s insuficijencijom rada srca. Srpski arhiv za celokupno lekarstvo. 2005 Jan;133(9-10):412-6.*

[22]*Jocić Stojanović J, Živković Z, Šumarac Dumanović M, Veković V. Kvalitet života gojazne dece sa astmom. Timocki Medicinski Glasnik. 2015 Oct 1;40(4).*
[23]*Gvozdenović B, Mitić S, Žugić V, Gvozdenović T A, Lazović N, Plavšić S. Odnos između stepena dispneje i kvaliteta života u vezi sa zdravljem bolesnika s hroničnom opstruktivnom bolešću pluća. Srpski arhiv za celokupno lekarstvo. 2007 Jan;135(9-10):547-53.*
[24]*Ursin H. Sensitization, somatization, and subjective health complaints. International journal of behavioral medicine. 1997 Jun;4:105-16.*
[25]*North CS, Hong BA, Alpers DH. Relationship of functional gastrointestinal disorders and psychiatric disorders: implications for treatment. World journal of gastroenterology: WJG. 2007 Apr 4;13(14):2020.*
[26]*Eriksen HR, Ursin H. Subjective health complaints, sensitization, and sustained cognitive activation (stress). Journal of psychosomatic research. 2004 Apr 1;56(4):445-8.*
[27]*Kulić L, Vujović M, Krstović SV, Jovanović J, Jovanović J. Examination of the impact of use of invasive cardiological procedures on quality of life of patients suffering from myocardial infarction. Zdravstvena zaštita. 2019;48(1):8-14.*
[28]*Garratt A, Schmidt L, Mackintosh A, Fitzpatrick R. Quality of life measurement: bibliographic study of patient assessed health outcome measures. Bmj. 2002 Jun 15;324(7351):1417.*
[29]*Theofilou P. Quality of life: definition and measurement. Europe's journal of psychology. 2013 Feb 1;9(1).*
[30]*Morris J, Perez D, McNoe B. The use of quality of life data in clinical practice. Quality of life research. 1997 Jan;7:85-91.*
[31]*Mooney A. Quality of life: Questionnaires and questions. Journal of health communication. 2006 Apr 1;11(3):327-41.*
[32]*Acquadro C, Conway K, Hareendran A, Aaronson N, European Regulatory Issues and Quality of Life Assessment (ERIQA) Group. Literature review of methods to translate health-related quality of life questionnaires for use in multinational clinical trials. Value in Health. 2008 May;11(3):509-21.*
[33]*Swaine-Verdier A, Doward LC, Hagell P, Thorsen H, McKenna SP. Adapting quality of life instruments. Value in health. 2004 Sep 1;7:S27-30.*
Haraldstad K, Wahl A, Andenæs R, Andersen JR, Andersen MH, Beisland E, Borge CR, Engebretsen E, Eisemann M, Halvorsrud L, Hanssen TA. A systematic review of quality of life research in medicine and health sciences. Quality of life Research. 2019 Oct;28:2641-50.

[34]Lee YT, Liu SI, Huang HC, Sun FJ, Huang CR, Yeung A. Validity and reliability of the Chinese version of the Short Form of Quality of Life Enjoyment and Satisfaction Questionnaire (Q-LES-Q-SF). Quality of Life Research. 2014 Apr;23:907-16.

[35]Stevanovic D. Quality of Life Enjoyment and Satisfaction Questionnaire–short form for quality of life assessments in clinical practice: A psychometric study. Journal of psychiatric and mental health nursing. 2011 Oct;18(8):744-50.

[36]Revicki DA, Kleinman L, Cella D. A history of health-related quality of life outcomes in psychiatry. Dialogues in clinical neuroscience. 2014 Jun 30;16(2):127-35.

[37]Michalak EE, Murray G, Levitt AJ, Levitan RD, Enns MW, Morehouse R, Tam EM, Cheung A, Lam RW. Quality of life as an outcome indicator in patients with seasonal affective disorder: results from the Can-SAD study. Psychological medicine. 2007 May;37(5):727-36.

[38]Riendeau RP, Sullivan JL, Meterko M, Stolzmann K, Williamson AK, Miller CJ, Kim B, Bauer MS. Factor structure of the Q-LES-Q short form in an enrolled mental health clinic population. Quality of Life Research. 2018 Nov;27:2953-64.

[39]Endicott J, Nee J, Harrison W, Blumenthal R. Quality of Life Enjoyment and Satisfaction Questionnaire: a new measure. Psychopharmacol Bull. 1993;29(2):321.

[40]WHO. WHOQOL-BREF: introduction, administration, scoring and generic version of the assessment: field trial version, December 1996: Geneva: World Health Organization; 1996.

[41]Norwood RJ. A review of etiologies of depression in COPD. Int J COPD. 2007;2(4):485–91.

[42]Martinez Rivera C, Costan Galicia J, Alcázar Navarrete B, Garcia-Polo C, Ruiz Iturriaga LA, Herrejón A, et al. Factors Associated with Depression in COPD: A Multicenter Study. Lung. Junio de 2016;194(3):335–43.

[43]Ivana Jelić, Goran Mihajlović, Filip Mihajlović, Nataša Minić, Miloš Ratinac and Maja Pantović-Stefanović, COPD and Depression Analysis in Regard to Obstructive Pulmonary Levels, Healthcare 2023, 11(8), 1175. https://doi.org/10.3390/healthcare11081175.

[44]Stage KB, Middelboe T, Stage TB, Sørensen CH. Depression in COPD – management and quality of life considerations. Int J Chron Obstruct Pulmon Dis. Septiembre de 2006;1(3):315–20.

[45]*Tønnesen P. Smoking cessation and COPD. European respiratory review. 2013 Mar 1;22(127):37-43.*
[46]*Bai JW, Chen XX, Liu S, Yu L, Xu JF. Smoking cessation affects the natural history of COPD. International journal of chronic obstructive pulmonary disease. 2017 Nov 16:3323-8.*
[47]*Fritzsche A, Clamor A, von Leupoldt A. Effects of medical and psychological treatment of depression in patients with COPD–a review. Respiratory medicine. 2011 Oct 1;105(10):1422-33.*
[48]*Yohannes AM, Alexopoulos GS. Depression and anxiety in patients with COPD. European Respiratory Review. 2014 Sep 1;23(133):345-9.*
[49]*Deb A, Sambamoorthi U. Depression treatment patterns among adults with chronic obstructive pulmonary disease and depression. Current medical research and opinion. 2017 Feb 1;33(2):201-8.*
[50]*Siraj RA, McKeever TM, Gibson JE, Bolton CE. Incidence of depression and antidepressant prescription in patients with COPD: A large UK population-based cohort study. Respiratory Medicine. 2022 May 1;196:106804.*
[51]*Buttery SC, Zysman M, Vikjord SA, Hopkinson NS, Jenkins C, Vanfleteren LE. Contemporary perspectives in COPD: patient burden, the role of gender and trajectories of multimorbidity. Respirology. 2021 May;26(5):419-41.*

4. Future Implications

Based on the literature review, it is believed that if the goal is to improve the efficiency and quality of treatment of patients, the assessment of quality of life should become an integral part of the practical, clinical and scientific research work of physicians of various specialties. There is great interest in the development of individual tests that measure the quality of life of patients with chronic diseases and depression. It is believed that quality of life is unique to each individual and that standard tests that require the selection of given answers cannot be adequately applied. The use of individual tests has immense value in clinical work, but it is limited in research due to the evaluation and summarization of results. For these reasons, numerous questions about the use of general and specific questionnaires in clinical work for the quality of life of the patient have remained unanswered. The answer to this question will be provided by the evolution of existing tests in further scientific research with an appropriate psychometric assessment of their impact on the patient's personality and their health status over time.

Selected Literature

1. Acquadro C, Conway K, Hareendran A, Aaronson N. European Regulatory Issues and Quality of Life Assessment (ERIQA) Group. Literature review of methods to translate health-related quality of life questionnaires for use in multinational clinical trials. Value in Health. 2008 May; 11(3): 509–21.
2. Adcock IM, Caramori G, Barnes PJ. Chronic obstructive pulmonary disease and lung cancer: New molecular insights. Respiration. 2011; 81(4): 265–84.
3. Afroz R, Hassan MN, Ibrahim NA. Review of air pollution and health impacts in Malaysia. Environmental research. 2003 Jun 1; 92(2): 71–7.
4. Agusti A, Gea J, Faner R. Biomarkers, the control panel and personalized COPD medicine. Respirology. 2016 Jan; 21(1): 24–33.
5. AIHW. Chronic Obstructive Pulmonary Disease (COPD). Cat. No. ACM 35. (Australian Institute of Health and Welfare, 2020).
6. Allison PJ, Locker D, Feine JS. Quality of life: a dynamic construct. Soc Sci Med. 1997; 45(2): 221–3
7. Akpinar K, Oğuzhanoğlu NK, Uğurlu TT. Efficacy of transcranial magnetic stimulation in treatment-resistant depression. Turkish Journal of Medical Sciences. 2022;52(4):1344-54.
8. Alqahtani JS, Njoku CM, Bereznicki B, Wimmer BC, Peterson GM, Kinsman L, Aldabayan YS, Alrajeh AM, Aldhahir AM, Mandal S, Hurst JR. Risk factors for all-cause hospital readmission following exacerbation of COPD: a systematic review and meta-analysis. Eur Respir Rev. 2020 Jun 3; 29(156): 190166. doi: 10.1183/16000617.0166-2019. PMID: 32499306.
9. An J, Zhou H, Yang T, Duan C, Bao C, Wan C, Shen Y, Wen F. Relationship of psychological factors with daily activities and quality of life in patients with chronic obstructive pulmonary disease in a Chinese rural population. Annals of palliative medicine. 2021 Feb 1; 10(2): 1675–84.
10. Annavarapu M, Mubeen T, Yaradesi N, Kantamneni P. A review on impact of mental health issues burden and its therapeutic strategies in COPD patients. 2021; 10(6): 396–409.
11. Antuni JD, Barnes PJ. Evaluation of individuals at risk for COPD: beyond the scope of the global initiative for chronic obstructive lung disease. Chronic Obstructive Pulmonary Diseases: Journal of the COPD Foundation. 2016; 3(3): 653–667.
12. APA. Depression Assessment Instruments. These instruments are relevant to the treatment of depression. 2023. Available at https://www.apa.org/depression-guideline/assessment

13. APA. The Economic Cost of Depression is Increasing; Direct Costs are Only a Small Part. 2021 May 27. Available at https://www.psychiatry.org/News-room/APA-Blogs/The-Economic-Cost-of-Depression-is-Increasing
14. Aria M, Misuraca M, Spano M. Mapping the evolution of social research and data science over 30 years of social indicators research. Social indicators research. 2020 Jun; 149: 803–31.
15. Arias-de la Torre J, Vilagut G, Ronaldson A, Serrano-Blanco A, Martín V, Peters M, Valderas JM, Dregan A, Alonso J. Prevalence and variability of current depressive disorder in 27 European countries: a population-based study. The Lancet Public Health. 2021 Oct 1; 6(10): e729–38.
16. Ayalon L, Goldfracht M, Bech P. 'Do you think you suffer from depression?' Reevaluating the use of a single item question for the screening of depression in older primary care patients. International Journal of Geriatric Psychiatry: A journal of the psychiatry of late life and allied sciences. 2010 May; 25(5): 497–502.
17. Bai JW, Chen XX, Liu S, Yu L, Xu JF. Smoking cessation affects the natural history of COPD. International journal of chronic obstructive pulmonary disease. 2017 Nov 16; 3323–8.
18. Balcells E, Gea J, Ferrer J, Serra I, Orozco-Levi M, de Batlle J, Rodriguez E, Benet M, Donaire-González D, Antó JM, Garcia-Aymerich J. Factors affecting the relationship between psychological status and quality of life in COPD patients. Health and quality of life outcomes. 2010 Dec; 8: 1–9.
19. Baraldo S, Turato G, Saetta M. Pathophysiology of the small airways in chronic obstructive pulmonary disease. Respiration. 2012; 84(2): 89–97.
20. Barnes PJ, Shapiro SD, Pauwels RA. Chronic obstructive pulmonary disease: molecular and cellular mechanisms. European Respiratory Journal. 2003 Oct 1; 22(4): 672–88.
21. Barnes PJ. Inflammatory mechanisms in patients with chronic obstructive pulmonary disease. Journal of Allergy and Clinical Immunology. 2016 Jul 1; 138(1): 16–27.
22. Batstra L, Bos EH, Neeleman J. Quantifying psychiatric comorbidity: Lessions from chronic disease epidemiology. Social psychiatry and psychiatric epidemiology. 2002 Mar; 37: 105–11.
23. Batut. Institut za javno zdravlje Srbije „Dr Milan Jovanović Batut“, Zdravstveno statistički godišnjak. Studija „Istraživanje zdravlja stanovništva Srbije 2019. godine“, 2019. Available at https://www.batut.org.rs/download/publikacije/ZdravljeStanovnistva2019.pdf
24. Batut. Institut za javno zdravlje Srbije „Dr Milan Jovanović Batut“, Zdravstveno statistički godišnjak. 2011.

25. Baxter AJ, Scott KM, Ferrari AJ, Norman RE, Vos T, Whiteford HA. Challenging the myth of an "epidemic" of common mental disorders: trends in the global prevalence of anxiety and depression between 1990 and 2010. Depression and anxiety. 2014 Jun; 31(6): 506–16.
26. Bellamy D, Smith J. Role of primary care in early diagnosis and effective management of COPD. International journal of clinical practice. 2007 Aug; 61(8): 1380–9.
27. Belvisi MG, Bottomley KM. The role of matrix metalloproteinases (MMPs) in the pathophysiology of chronic obstructive pulmonary disease (COPD): a therapeutic role for inhibitors of MMPs? Inflammation research. 2003 Mar; 52: 95–100.
28. Benowitz NL, Hatsukami D. Gender differences in the pharmacology of nicotine addiction. Addiction biology. Oct 1998; 3(4): 383–404.
29. Billings AG, Moos RH. Comparisons of children of depressed and nondepressed parents: A social-environmental perspective. Journal of Abnormal Child Psychology. 1983 Dec; 11: 463–85.
30. Borthwick-Duffy SA. Quality of life and quality of care in mental retardation. Mental retardation in the year 2000. Berlin: Ed. L. Rowitz; 1992; 52–66.
31. Bozkurt N, Bozkurt Aİ, Dirol H. Anxiety/depression scores and affecting factors in COPD patients. Eurasian Journal of Pulmonology. 2022; 24(2): 122–129.
32. Brashier BB, Kodgule R. Risk factors and pathophysiology of chronic obstructive pulmonary disease (COPD). J Assoc Physicians India. 2012 Feb 1; 60(Suppl): 17–21.
33. Bromet E, Andrade LH, Hwang I, Sampson NA, Alonso J, De Girolamo G, De Graaf R, Demyttenaere K, Hu C, Iwata N, Karam AN. Cross-national epidemiology of DSM-IV major depressive episode. BMC medicine. 2011 Dec; 9(1): 1–6.
34. Brown J, Cohen P, Johnson JG, Smailes EM. Childhood abuse and neglect: specificity of effects on adolescent and young adult depression and suicidality. Journal of the American Academy of Child & Adolescent Psychiatry. 1999 Dec 1; 38(12): 1490–6.
35. Burney P, Jithoo A, Koto B, et al. Chronic obstructive pulmonary disease mortality and prevalence: the associations with smoking and poverty-a BOLD analysis. Thorax 2014; 69(5): 465–473.
36. Buttery SC, Zysman M, Vikjord SA, Hopkinson NS, Jenkins C, Vanfleteren LE. Contemporary perspectives in COPD: patient burden, the role of gender and trajectories of multimorbidity. Respirology. 2021 May; 26(5): 419–41.

37. Cafarella PA, Effing TW, Usmani ZA, Frith PA. Treatments for anxiety and depression in patients with chronic obstructive pulmonary disease: a literature review. Respirology. 2012 May; 17(4): 627–38.
38. Cavaillès A, Brinchault-Rabin G, Dixmier A et al. Comorbidities of COPD. Eur Resp Rev. 2013; 22: 454–475. doi: 10.1183/09059180.00008612
39. Chanques G, Constantin JM, Devlin JW, Ely EW, Fraser GL, Gélinas C, Girard TD, Guérin C, Jabaudon M, Jaber S, Mehta S. Analgesia and sedation in patients with ARDS. Intensive care medicine. 2020 Dec; 46: 2342–56.
40. Cohen BH, Ball Jr WC, Brashears S, Diamond EL, Kreiss P, Levy DA, Menkes HA, Permutt S, Tockman MS. Risk factors in chronic obstructive pulmonary disease (COPD). American journal of epidemiology. 1977 Mar 1; 105(3): 223–32.
41. Collins PF, Stratton RJ, Elia M. Nutritional support in chronic obstructive pulmonary disease: a systematic review and meta-analysis. Am J Clin Nutr. 2012 Jun; 95(6): 1385–1395.
42. Cougle JR, Timpano KR, Sachs-Ericsson N, Keough ME, Riccardi CJ. Examining the unique relationships between anxiety disorders and childhood physical and sexual abuse in the National Comorbidity Survey Replication. Psychiatry research. 2010 May 15; 177(1-2): 150–5.
43. Crisafulli E, Costi S, Luppi F, Cirelli G, Cilione C, Coletti O, Fabbri LM, Clini EM. Role of comorbidities in a cohort of patients with COPD undergoing pulmonary rehabilitation. Thorax. Jun 1, 2008; 63(6): 487–92.
44. Cummnins RA. Objective and subjective quality of life: an interactive model. Soc Indic Res. 2000; 52(1): 55–72.
45. Čekerevac I. Sistemski efekti hronične opstruktivne bolesti pluća. Doktorska disertacija, Kragujevac, 2010.
46. Daly M. Prevalence of depression among adolescents in the US from 2009 to 2019: analysis of trends by sex, race/ethnicity, and income. Journal of Adolescent Health. 2022 Mar 1; 70(3): 496–9.
47. Deb A, Sambamoorthi U. Depression treatment patterns among adults with chronic obstructive pulmonary disease and depression. Current medical research and opinion. 2017 Feb 1; 33(2): 201–8.
48. Di Rosanna P, Salvatore C. Reactive oxygen species, inflammation, and lung diseases. Current pharmaceutical design. 2012 Sep 1; 18(26): 3889–900.
49. Dome P, Lazary J, Kalapos MP, Rihmer Z. Smoking, nicotine and neuropsychiatric disorders. Neuroscience & Biobehavioral Reviews. 2010 Feb 1; 34(3): 295–342.

50. Drummond MB, Buist AS, Crapo JD, Wise RA, Rennard SI. Chronic obstructive pulmonary disease: NHLBI workshop on the primary prevention of chronic lung diseases. Annals of the American Thoracic Society. 2014 Apr; 11(Supplement 3): S154–60.
51. Dua R, Das A, Kumar A, Kumar S, Mishra M, Sharma K. Association of comorbid anxiety and depression with chronic obstructive pulmonary disease. Lung India 2018; 35: 31–6.
52. Dugalić S. Značaj sporta i ponašanja sportista za formiranje stavova ljudi. SPORT-Nauka i Praksa, 5. 2016; 5–22.
53. Durstine JL, Gordon B, Wang Z, Luo X. Chronic disease and the link to physical activity. Journal of sport and health science. 2013 Mar 1; 2(1): 3–11.
54. Eapen MS, Hansbro PM, Larsson-Callerfelt AK, Jolly MK, Myers S, Sharma P, Jones B, Rahman MA, Markos J, Chia C, Larby J. Chronic obstructive pulmonary disease and lung cancer: underlying pathophysiology and new therapeutic modalities. Drugs. 2018 Nov; 78: 1717–40.
55. ECDC. European Centre for Disease Prevention and Control. 2023. https://www.ecdc.europa.eu/en
56. Endicott J, Nee J, Harrison W, Blumenthal R. Quality of Life Enjoyment and Satisfaction Questionnaire: a new measure. Psychopharmacol Bull. 1993; 29(2): 321–326.
57. Eriksen HR, Ursin H. Subjective health complaints, sensitization, and sustained cognitive activation (stress). Journal of psychosomatic research. 2004 Apr 1; 56(4): 445–8.
58. Fan VS, Ramsey SD, Giardino ND, Make BJ, Emery CF, Diaz PT, Benditt JO, Mosenifar Z, McKenna R, Curtis JL, Fishman AP. Sex, depression, and risk of hospitalization and mortality in chronic obstructive pulmonary disease. Archives of internal medicine. 2007 Nov 26; 167(21): 2345–53.
59. Felce D, Perry J. Quality of life: its definition and measurement. Res Dev Disabil.1995; 16(1): 51–74.
60. Fritzsche A, Clamor A, von Leupoldt A. Effects of medical and psychological treatment of depression in patients with COPD–a review. Respiratory medicine. 2011 Oct 1; 105(10): 1422–33.
61. Fuhrer R, Wessely S. The epidemiology of fatigue and depression: a French primary-care study. Psychological medicine. 1995 Sep; 25(5): 895–905.
62. Furutate R, Ishii T, Motegi T, Hattori K, Kusunoki Y, Gemma A, Kida K. The neutrophil to lymphocyte ratio is related to disease severity and exacerbation in patients with chronic obstructive pulmonary disease. Internal Medicine. 2016; 55(3): 223–9.

63. Garratt A, Schmidt L, Mackintosh A, Fitzpatrick R. Quality of life measurement: bibliographic study of patient assessed health outcome measures. Bmj. 2002 Jun 15; 324(7351): 1417.
64. Gatchel RJ. Comorbidity of chronic pain and mental health disorders: the biopsychosocial perspective. American Psychologist. 2004 Nov; 59(8): 795.
65. GOLD 2013. Global Initiative for Chronic Obstructive Lung Disease (GOLD) 2013. Available at http://www.goldcopd.org/
66. GOLD 2023. Global Initiative For Chronic Obstructive Lung Diseases. 2023 Report. Available at https://goldcopd.org/2023-gold-report-2/
67. GOLD 2021. Global Strategy for the Diagnosis, Management and Prevention of Chronic Obstructive Pulmonary Disease: 2021 Report. Available at https://goldcopd.org/wp-content/uploads/2020/11/GOLD-REPORT-2021-v1.1-25Nov20_WMV.pdf. Accessed: July 26, 2021.
68. GOLD 2018. Global Strategy for the Diagnosis, Management, and Prevention of Chronic Obstructive Pulmonary Disease. Updated 2018. http://www.goldcopd.org. Available at https://goldcopd.org/wp-content/uploads/2017/11/GOLD-2018-v6.0-FINAL-revised-20-Nov_WMS.pdf
69. Goldenberg DL. Diagnosis and differential diagnosis of fibromyalgia. The American journal of medicine. 2009 Dec 1; 122(12): S14–21.
70. Graumam RQ, Pinheiro MM, Nery LE, Castro CH. Increased rate of osteoporosis, low lean mass, and fragility fractures in COPD patients: association with disease severity. Osteoporosis International. 2018 Jun; 29: 1457–68.
71. Gray C, Ambady L, Chao S, Smith W, Yoon J. Virtual Management of Chronic Conditions During the COVID-19 Pandemic: Insights From Primary Care Providers and Clinical Pharmacists. Military Medicine. 2023 Jul 1; 188(7-8): e2615–20.
72. Greenberg PE, Fournier AA, Sisitsky T, Pike CT, Kessler RC. The economic burden of adults with major depressive disorder in the United States (2005 and 2010). The Journal of clinical psychiatry. 2015 Feb 25; 76(2): 5356.
73. Greenberg PE, Fournier AA, Sisitsky T, Simes M, Berman R, Koenigsberg SH, Kessler RC. The economic burden of adults with major depressive disorder in the United States (2010 and 2018). Pharmacoeconomics. 2021 Jun; 39(6): 653–65. Available at https://pubmed.ncbi.nlm.nih.gov/33950419/
74. Gruenberg AM, Goldstein RD, Pincus HA. Classification of depression: Research and diagnostic criteria: DSM-IV and ICD-10. Biology of depression: From novel insights to therapeutic strategies. 2005 Jan 26: 1–2.
75. Gvozdenović B, Mitić S, Žugić V, Gvozdenović TA, Lazović N, Plavšić S. Odnos između stepena dispneje i kvaliteta života u vezi sa zdravljem

bolesnika s hroničnom opstruktivnom bolešću pluća. Srpski arhiv za celokupno lekarstvo. 2007 Jan; 135(9-10): 547–53.

76. Hall A. Quality of life and value assessment in health care. Health Care Analysis. 2020 Mar; 28(1): 45–61.

77. Hamilton J, Guthrie E, Creed F, Thompson D, Tomenson B, Bennett R, Moriarty K, Stephens W, Liston R. A randomized controlled trial of psychotherapy in patients with chronic functional dyspepsia. Gastroenterology. 2000 Sep 1; 119(3): 661–9.

78. Haraldstad K, Wahl A, Andenæs R, Andersen JR, Andersen MH, Beisland E, Borge CR, Engebretsen E, Eisemann M, Halvorsrud L, Hanssen TA. A systematic review of quality of life research in medicine and health sciences. Quality of life Research. 2019 Oct; 28: 2641–50.

79. Hardin M, Silverman EK. Chronic obstructive pulmonary disease genetics: a review of the past and a look into the future. Chronic Obstructive Pulmonary Diseases: Journal of the COPD Foundation. 2014; 1(1): 33.

80. Hardinge M, Annandale J, Bourne S, Cooper B, Evans A, Freeman D, Green A, Hippolyte S, Knowles V, MacNee W, McDonnell L. British Thoracic Society guidelines for home oxygen use in adults: accredited by NICE. Thorax. 2015 Jun 1; 70(Suppl 1): i1–43.

81. Hikichi M, Mizumura K, Maruoka S, Gon Y. Pathogenesis of chronic obstructive pulmonary disease (COPD) induced by cigarette smoke. Journal of thoracic disease. 2019 Oct; 11(Suppl 17): S2129.

82. Hiller AM, Piitulainen E, Jehpsson L, Tanash H. Decline in FEV1 and hospitalized exacerbations in individuals with severe alpha-1 antitrypsin deficiency. International journal of chronic obstructive pulmonary disease. 2019 May 23: 1075–83.

83. Hogea SP, Tudorache E, Fildan AP, Fira-Mladinescu O, Marc M, Oancea C. Risk factors of chronic obstructive pulmonary disease exacerbations. Clin Respir J. 2020; 14(3): 183–197. doi:10.1111/crj.13129.

84. Ibrahim AK, Kelly SJ, Adams CE, Glazebrook C. A systematic review of studies of depression prevalence in university students. Journal of psychiatric research. 2013 Mar 1; 47(3): 391–400.

85. Jaffe DH, Rive B, Denee TR. The humanistic and economic burden of treatment-resistant depression in Europe: a cross-sectional study. BMC psychiatry. 2019 Dec; 19: 1-1.

86. Jain D, Chaudhary P, Varshney N, Bin Razzak KS, Verma D, Khan Zahra TR, Janmeda P, Sharifi-Rad J, Daştan SD, Mahmud S, Docea AO. Tobacco smoking and liver cancer risk: potential avenues for carcinogenesis. Journal of Oncology. 2021 Dec 10.

87. Ivana Jelić, Goran Mihajlović, Jovanka Kos, Učestalost simptoma depresije i depresivne epizode u primarnoj zdravstvenoj zaštiti, Engrami 2013; 35(1):5-11.
88. Jelić I, Mihajlović G, Mihajlović F, Minić N, Ratinac M, Pantović-Stefanović M. COPD and Depression Analysis in Regard to Obstructive Pulmonary Levels. In Healthcare. 2023 Apr 19 (Vol. 11, No. 8, p. 1175). MDPI.
89. Ivana Jelić, Goran Mihajlović, Miloš Ratinac, Katarina Mihajlović, Sara Mijailović and Ivan Cekerevac, Psychophysical and Social Functioning of Patients with Chronic Obstructive Lung Disease and Depression, Eur. J. Investig. Health Psychol. Educ. 2023, 13, 2841–2852. https://doi.org/10.3390/ejihpe13120196.
90. Ivana Jelić, Marko Folić, Filip Mihajlović, Slobodan Janković, Goran Mihajlović, The effects of antidepressant therapy on health-related quality of life in patients with a chronic obstructive pulmonary disease and depressive symptoms, Serbian Journal of experimental and Clinical Research 2021; doi: 10.2478/sjecr-2021-0068.
91. Jocić Stojanović J, Živković Z, Šumarac Dumanović M, Veković V. Kvalitet života gojazne dece sa astmom. Timocki Medicinski Glasnik. 2015 Oct 1; 40(4).
92. Johnston KM, Powell LC, Anderson IM, Szabo S, Cline S. The burden of treatment-resistant depression: a systematic review of the economic and quality of life literature. Journal of affective disorders. 2019 Jan 1; 242: 195–210.
93. Katon W, Ciechanowski P. Impact of major depression on chronic medical illness. Journal of psychosomatic research. 2002 Oct 1; 53(4): 859–63.
94. Katz IR. On the inseparability of mental and physical health in aged persons: lessons from depression and medical comorbidity. The American Journal of Geriatric Psychiatry. 1996 Dec 1; 4(1): 1–6.
95. Keller MB, McCullough JP, Klein DN, Arnow B, Dunner DL, Gelenberg AJ, Markowitz JC, Nemeroff CB, Russell JM, Thase ME, Trivedi MH. A comparison of nefazodone, the cognitive behavioral-analysis system of psychotherapy, and their combination for the treatment of chronic depression. New England journal of medicine. 2000 May 18; 342(20): 1462–70.
96. Keshavarz K, Hedayati A, Rezaei M, Goudarzi Z, Moghimi E, Rezaee M, Lotfi F. Economic burden of major depressive disorder: a case study in Southern Iran. BMC psychiatry. 2022 Aug 30; 22(1): 577.
97. Kim KU, Park HK, Jung HY, Ahn JJ, Moon E, Kim YS, Lee MK, Lee H. Association of depression with disease severity in patients with chronic obstructive pulmonary disease. Lung. 2014 Apr; 192: 243–9.

98. Kimmel PL, Weihs K, Peterson RA. Survival in hemodialysis patients: the role of depression. Journal of the American Society of Nephrology. 1993 Jul 1; 4(1): 12–27.
99. Kirkham PA, Barnes PJ. Oxidative stress in COPD. Chest. 2013 Jul 1; 144(1): 266–73.
100. Kiros F, Shakya KM, Rupakheti M, Regmi RP, Maharjan R, Byanju RM, Naja M, Mahata K, Kathayat B, Peltier RE. Variability of anthropogenic gases: Nitrogen oxides, sulfur dioxide, ozone and ammonia in Kathmandu Valley, Nepal. Aerosol and Air Quality Research. 2016 Dec; 16(12): 3088–101.
101. Krabbe PF. Thurstone scaling as a measurement method to quantify subjective health outcomes. Medical care. 2008 Apr 1: 357–65.
102. Kulić L, Vujović M, Krstović SV, Jovanović J, Jovanović J. Examination of the impact of use of invasive cardiological procedures on quality of life of patients suffering from myocardial infarction. Zdravstvena zaštita. 2019; 48(1): 8–14.
103. Lacasse Y, Rousseau L, Maltais F. Prevalence of depressive symptoms and depression in patients with severe oxygen-dependent chronic obstructive pulmonary disease. Journal of Cardiopulmonary Rehabilitation and Prevention. 2001 Mar 1; 21(2): 80–6.
104. LaGrant B, Marquis BO, Berg AT, Grinspan ZM. Depression and anxiety in children with epilepsy and other chronic health conditions: national estimates of prevalence and risk factors. Epilepsy & Behavior. 2020 Feb 1; 103: 106828.
105. Lamprecht B, McBurnie MA, Vollmer WM, et al.COPD in never smokers: results from the population-based burden of obstructive lung disease study. Chest, 2011; 139(4): 752–63.
106. Lazic Z, Stankovic I, Milenkovic B, Zvezdin B, Hromis S, Jankovic S, et al. Characteristics of COPD Phenotypes in Serbia. Int J Chron Obstruct Pulmon Dis. 2021; 16: 643–54.
107. Lee YT, Liu SI, Huang HC, Sun FJ, Huang CR, Yeung A. Validity and reliability of the Chinese version of the Short Form of Quality of Life Enjoyment and Satisfaction Questionnaire (Q-LES-Q-SF). Quality of Life Research. 2014 Apr; 23: 907–16.
108. Lépine JP, Briley M. The increasing burden of depression. Neuropsychiatric disease and treatment. 2011 May 31; 7(Suppl1): 3–7.
109. Likert R. A technique for the measurement of attitudes. Archives of psychology. 1932.

110. Lim SU, Lee EH, Hwang ST, Hong SH, Kim JH. The beck depression inventory: psychometric properties in Korean adult populations. Korean Journal of Clinical Psychology. 2019 Aug; 38(3): 300–7.
111. Lin P, Campbell DG, Chaney EF, Liu CF, Heagerty P, Felker BL, Hedrick SC. The influence of patient preference on depression treatment in primary care. Annals of Behavioral Medicine. 2005 Oct 1; 30(2): 164–73.
112. Liu D, Meister M, Zhang S, Vong CI, Wang S, Fang R, Li L, Wang PG, Massion P, Ji X. Identification of lipid biomarker from serum in patients with chronic obstructive pulmonary disease. Respiratory Research. 2020 Dec; 21: 1–3.
113. Liu Y, Tang X. Depressive syndromes in autoimmune disorders of the nervous system: prevalence, etiology, and influence. Frontiers in psychiatry. 2018 Sep 25; 9: 451.
114. Loi AT, Hoonhorst SJ, Franciosi L, Bischoff R, Hoffmann RF, Heijink I, van Oosterhout AJ, Boezen HM, Timens W, Postma DS, Lammers JW. Acute and chronic inflammatory responses induced by smoking in individuals susceptible and non-susceptible to development of COPD: from specific disease phenotyping towards novel therapy. Protocol of a cross-sectional study. Bmj Open. 2013 Jan 1; 3(2): e002178.
115. Long J, Ouyang Y, Duan H, Xiang Z, Ma H, Ju M, Sun D. Multiple factor analysis of depression and/or anxiety in patients with acute exacerbation chronic obstructive pulmonary disease. International Journal of Chronic Obstructive Pulmonary Disease. 2020 Jun 19: 1449–64.
116. López-Campos JL, Tan W, Soriano JB. Global burden of COPD. Respirology. 2016 Jan; 21(1): 14–23.
117. Lou P, Zhu Y, Chen P, Zhang P, Yu J, Wang Y, Chen N, Zhang L, Wu H, Zhao J. Interaction of depressive and anxiety symptoms on the mortality of patients with COPD: a preliminary study. COPD: Journal of Chronic Obstructive Pulmonary Disease. 2014 Aug 1; 11(4): 444–50.
118. Löwe B, Gräfe K, Zipfel S, Witte S, Loerch B, Herzog W. Diagnosing ICD-10 depressive episodes: superior criterion validity of the Patient Health Questionnaire. Psychotherapy and psychosomatics. 2004; 73(6): 386–90.
119. Maharaj S, Lees T, Lal S. Prevalence and risk factors of depression, anxiety, and stress in a cohort of Australian nurses. International journal of environmental research and public health. 2019 Jan; 16(1): 61.
120. Manea L, Gilbody S, McMillan D. Optimal cut-off score for diagnosing depression with the Patient Health Questionnaire (PHQ-9): a meta-analysis. Cmaj. 2012 Feb 21; 184(3): E191–6.

121. Markowitz S, Friedman MA, Arent SM. Understanding the relation between obesity and depression: causal mechanisms and implications for treatment. Clinical Psychology: Science and Practice. 2008 Mar; 15(1): 1.
122. Marsh S, Aldington S, Shirtcliffe P, Weatherall M, Beasley R. Smoking and COPD: what really are the risks? Eur. Respir. J. 2006; 28: 883–886.
123. Martinez CH, Mannino DM, Divo MJ. Defining COPD-related comorbidities, 2004-2014. J COPD F. 2014; 1(1): 51–63.
124. Martinez Rivera C, Costan Galicia J, Alcázar Navarrete B, Garcia-Polo C, Ruiz Iturriaga LA, Herrejón A, et al. Factors Associated with Depression in COPD: A Multicenter Study. Lung. Junio de 2016; 194(3): 335–43.
125. Martinović I. Pet odsto stanovništva Srbije u depresiji. 12. februar 2019. 2019. Available at https://www.slobodnaevropa.org/a/pet-odsto-stanovnistva-srbije-u-depresiji/29764316.html
126. Maurer J, Rebbapragada V, Borson S, Goldstein R, Kunik ME, Yohannes AM, Hanania NA. Anxiety and depression in COPD: current understanding, unanswered questions, and research needs. Chest. 2008 Oct 1; 134(4): 43S–56S.
127. Michalak EE, Murray G, Levitt AJ, Levitan RD, Enns MW, Morehouse R, Tam EM, Cheung A, Lam RW. Quality of life as an outcome indicator in patients with seasonal affective disorder: results from the Can-SAD study. Psychological medicine. 2007 May; 37(5): 727–36.
128. Ministarstvo zdravlja i socijalne zaštite Republike Srpske. Klinički vodič - Duševni poremećaji i poremećaji ponašanja. 2008. Available at https://www.vladars.net/sr-SP-Cyrl/Vlada/Ministarstva/MZSZ/Documents/depresija_distimija.pdf
129. Ministarstvo zdravlja Republike Srbije. 2011. Nacionalni vodič dobre kliničke prakse. Depresija [orig. Национални водич добре клиничке праксе. Депресија]. Available at https://www.zdravlje.gov.rs/view_file.php?file_id=675&cache=sr
130. Mold E. The Prevalance of Depression amongst People with Chronic Obstructive Pulmonary Disease on Long Term Oxygen Therapy. 2010.
131. Moll M, Sakornsakolpat P, Shrine N, Hobbs BD, DeMeo DL, John C, Guyatt AL, McGeachie MJ, Gharib SA, Obeidat ME, Lahousse L. Chronic obstructive pulmonary disease and related phenotypes: polygenic risk scores in population-based and case-control cohorts. The Lancet Respiratory Medicine. 2020 Jul 1; 8(7): 696–708.
132. Mooney A. Quality of life: Questionnaires and questions. Journal of health communication. 2006 Apr 1; 11(3): 327–41.

133. Morin Amy LCSW. 2021. Screening for Depression: How Depression Tests Work. May 28, 2021. Available at https://www.verywellmind.com/depression-tests-mood-disorder-4174922
134. Morris J, Perez D, McNoe B. The use of quality of life data in clinical practice. Quality of life research. 1997 Jan; 7: 85–91.
135. Mount BM, Cohen SR. Quality of life in the face of life-threatening illnes: What should we be measuring? Current Oncology 1995; 2: 121–25.
136. NCHC. National Center for Health Statistics. 2023. Antidepressant Use Among Adults: United States, 2015-2018. Available at https://www.cdc.gov/nchs/products/databriefs/db377.htm
137. NCHC. National Center for Health Statistics. 2023. Depression. Available at https://www.cdc.gov/nchs/fastats/depression.htm
138. NCHC. National Center for Health Statistics. 2023. Depression. Morbidity. Available at https://www.cdc.gov/nchs/data/nhis/earlyrelease/EarlyRelease202009-508.pdf
139. NCHC. National Center for Health Statistics. 2023. National Ambulatory Medical Care Survey: 2019 National Summary Tables. Available at https://www.cdc.gov/nchs/data/ahcd/namcs_summary/2019-namcs-web-tables-508.pdf
140. Nemeroff CB, Heim CM, Thase ME, Klein DN, Rush AJ, Schatzberg AF, Ninan PT, McCullough Jr JP, Weiss PM, Dunner DL, Rothbaum BO. Differential responses to psychotherapy versus pharmacotherapy in patients with chronic forms of major depression and childhood trauma. Proceedings of the National Academy of Sciences. 2003 Nov 25; 100(24): 14293–6.
141. North CS, Hong BA, Alpers DH. Relationship of functional gastrointestinal disorders and psychiatric disorders: implications for treatment. World journal of gastroenterology: WJG. 2007 Apr 4; 13(14): 2020.
142. Norwood RJ. A review of etiologies of depression in COPD. Int J COPD. 2007; 2(4): 485–91.
143. Obeid S, Azzi V, Hallit S. Validation and psychometric properties of the Arabic version of Hamilton Depression Rating Scale 7 items (HAMD-7) among non-clinical and clinical samples of Lebanese adults. Plos one. 2023 May 18; 18(5): e0285665.
144. O'Boyle C. The Schedule for the evaluation of individual Quality of life (SEI-QOL). Int J Ment Health. 1994; 23(3): 3–23.
145. O'Connor EA, Whitlock EP, Gaynes B, Beil TL. Screening for depression in adults and older adults in primary care: an updated systematic review. Available at https://www.ncbi.nlm.nih.gov/books/NBK36410/
146. Oswald-Mammosser M, Weitzenblum E, Quoix E, Moser G, Chaouat A, Charpentier C, Kessler R. Prognostic factors in COPD patients receiving

long-term oxygen therapy: importance of pulmonary artery pressure. Chest. 1995 May 1; 107(5): 1193–8.
147. Pedrozo-Pupo JC, Campo-Arias A, Ceballos-Ospino GA. Quality of life and depression in COPD patients in the Colombian Caribbean. The Clinical Respiratory Journal. 2021 Sep; 15(9): 944–8.
148. Peterson JB. Maps of meaning: The architecture of belief. Routledge; 2002 Sep 11.
149. Polsky D, Doshi JA, Marcus S, Oslin D, Rothbard A, Thomas N, Thompson CL. Long-term risk for depressive symptoms after a medical diagnosis. Archives of internal medicine. 2005 Jun 13; 165(11): 1260–6.
150. Pravno informacioni sistem Repblike Srbije. Program o zaštiti mentalnog zdravlja u Republici Srbiji za period 2019–2026. godine. „Službeni glasnik RS", broj 84 od 29. novembra 2019. 2019. Available at https://www.pravno-informacioni-sistem.rs/SlGlasnikPortal/eli/rep/sgrs/vlada/drugiakt/2019/84/1
151. Rabe KF, Hurd S, Anzueto A, Barnes PJ, Buist SA, Calverley P, Fukuchi Y, Jenkins C, Rodriguez-Roisin R, Van Weel C, Zielinski J. Global strategy for the diagnosis, management, and prevention of chronic obstructive pulmonary disease: GOLD executive summary. American journal of respiratory and critical care medicine. 2007 Sep 15; 176(6): 532–55.
152. Radovanović N, Jakovljević Đ, Kanjuh V. Quality of life after open heart surgery: a ten year follow-up research study. U: Kanjuh V, Radovanović N, eds. Atherothrombotic coronary heart disease: morphological-clinical correlations. Belgrade: Serbian Academy of Sciences and Arts; 2008.
153. Revicki DA, Kleinman L, Cella D. A history of health-related quality of life outcomes in psychiatry. Dialogues in clinical neuroscience. 2014 Jun 30; 16(2): 127–35.
154. Riendeau RP, Sullivan JL, Meterko M, Stolzmann K, Williamson AK, Miller CJ, Kim B, Bauer MS. Factor structure of the Q-LES-Q short form in an enrolled mental health clinic population. Quality of Life Research. 2018 Nov; 27: 2953–64.
155. Ristić Ž. Objedinjavanje kvantitativnih i kvalitativnih istraživanja. Beograd: Evropski centar za mir i razvoj – Univerzitet za mir Ujedinjenih nacija. 2016.
156. Rizzo R, Piccinelli M, Mazzi MA, Bellantuono C, Tansella M. The Personal Health Questionnaire: a new screening instrument for detection of ICD-10 depressive disorders in primary care. Psychological Medicine. 2000 Jul; 30(4): 831–40.
157. Schalock R. Three decades of quality of life. Focus Autism Other Dev Disabl. 2000; 15(2): 116–27.

158. Schramm E, Kriston L, Elsaesser M, Fangmeier T, Meister R, Bausch P, Zobel I, Bailer J, Wambach K, Backenstrass M, Klein JP. Two-year follow-up after treatment with the cognitive behavioral analysis system of psychotherapy versus supportive psychotherapy for early-onset chronic depression. Psychotherapy and psychosomatics. 2019; 88(3): 154–64.
159. Seersholm N, Kok-Jensen A, Dirksen A. Decline in FEV1 among patients with severe hereditary alpha 1-antitrypsin deficiency type PiZ. American journal of respiratory and critical care medicine. 1995 Dec; 152(6): 1922–5.
160. Sekine Y, Katsura H, Koh E, Hiroshima K, Fujisawa T. Early detection of COPD is important for lung cancer surveillance. European Respiratory Journal. 2012 May 1; 39(5): 1230–40.
161. Siniscalchi KA, Broome ME, Fish J, Ventimiglia J, Thompson J, Roy P, Pipes R, Trivedi M. Depression screening and measurement-based care in primary care. Journal of primary care & community health. 2020 Nov; 11:2150132720931261. Available at https://www.ncbi.nlm.nih.gov/pmc/articles/PMC7673056/
162. Siraj RA, McKeever TM, Gibson JE, Bolton CE. Incidence of depression and antidepressant prescription in patients with COPD: A large UK population-based cohort study. Respiratory Medicine. 2022 May 1; 196: 106804.
163. Sirgy MJ. The psychology of quality of life: Wellbeing and positive mental health. Social Indicators Research Series. Springer International Publishing, Cham. https://doi. org/10.1007/978-3-030-71888-6. 2021.
164. Shahid A, Wilkinson K, Marcu S, Shapiro CM. Hamilton Rating Scale for Depression (HAM-D). InSTOP, THAT and One Hundred Other Sleep Scales 2011 Nov 24 (pp. 187-190). New York, NY: Springer New York.
165. Solé B, Verdolini N, Amoretti S, Montejo L, Rosa AR, Hogg B, Garcia-Rizo C, Mezquida G, Bernardo M, Martinez-Aran A, Vieta E. Effects of the COVID-19 pandemic and lockdown in Spain: comparison between community controls and patients with a psychiatric disorder. Preliminary results from the BRIS-MHC STUDY. Journal of affective disorders. 2021 Feb 15; 281: 13–23.
166. Stage KB, Middelboe T, Stage TB, Sørensen CH. Depression in COPD – management and quality of life considerations. Int J Chron Obstruct Pulmon Dis. Septiembre de 2006; 1(3): 315–20.
167. Stevanovic D. Quality of Life Enjoyment and Satisfaction Questionnaire–short form for quality of life assessments in clinical practice: A psychometric study. Journal of psychiatric and mental health nursing. 2011 Oct; 18(8): 744–50.

168. Stoller JK, Aboussouan LS. Alpha1-antitrypsin deficiency. Lancet. 2005; 365(9478): 2225–36.
169. Story DA, Tait AR. Survey research. Anesthesiology. 2019 Feb; 130(2): 192–202.
170. Sundh J, Ställberg B, Lisspers K, Montgomery SM, Janson C. Co-morbidity, body mass index and quality of life in COPD using the Clinical COPD Questionnaire. COPD: Journal of Chronic Obstructive Pulmonary Disease. 2011 May 27; 8(3): 173–81.
171. Swaine-Verdier A, Doward LC, Hagell P, Thorsen H, McKenna SP. Adapting quality of life instruments. Value in health. 2004 Sep 1; 7: S27–30.
172. Terzić Z, Bjegović V, Marinković J, Draganić G, Ljubić B, Seferović J. Merenje kvaliteta života bolesnika s insuficijencijom rada srca. Srpski arhiv za celokupno lekarstvo. 2005 Jan; 133(9-10): 412–6.
173. Theofilou P. Quality of life: definition and measurement. Europe's journal of psychology. 2013 Feb 1; 9(1).
174. Thurstone LL. A law of comparative judgments. Psychol Rev. 1927; 34: 273–286.
175. Tønnesen P. Smoking cessation and COPD. European respiratory review. 2013 Mar 1; 22(127): 37–43.
176. Trivić B. Analiza troškova nastalih hospitalizacijom u tercijarnoj ustanovi usled akutnih egzacerbacija hronične opstruktivne bolesti pluća. Univerzitet u Novom Sadu. 2016 May 23.
177. Tselebis A, Kosmas E, Bratis D, Moussas G, Karkanias A, Ilias I, Siafakas N, Vgontzas A, Tzanakis N. Prevalence of alexithymia and its association with anxiety and depression in a sample of Greek chronic obstructive pulmonary disease (COPD) outpatients. Annals of General Psychiatry. 2010 Dec; 9(1): 1–7.
178. Tselebis A, Pachi A, Ilias I, Kosmas E, Bratis D, Moussas G, Tzanakis N. Strategies to improve anxiety and depression in patients with COPD: a mental health perspective. Neuropsychiatric disease and treatment. 2016 Feb 9: 297–328.
179. U.S. Department of Health and Human Services. The Health Consequences of Smoking— 50 Years of Progress: A Report of the Surgeon General. Atlanta: U.S. Department of Health and Human Services, Centers for Disease Control and Prevention, National Center for Chronic Disease Prevention and Health Promotion, Office on Smoking and Health, 2014.
180. Umareta NR. A Literature Review of Depression and Anxiety in Chronic Obstructive Pulmonary Disease (COPD) Patients. Scientia Psychiatrica. 2023; 4(1): 339–45.

181. Ursin H. Sensitization, somatization, and subjective health complaints. International journal of behavioral medicine. 1997 Jun; 4: 105–16.
182. Urtasun M, Daray FM, Teti GL, Coppolillo F, Herlax G, Saba G, Rubinstein A, Araya R, Irazola V. Validation and calibration of the patient health questionnaire (PHQ-9) in Argentina. BMC psychiatry. 2019 Dec; 19(1): 1–0.
183. Van de Velde S, Bracke P, Levecque K. Gender differences in depression in 23 European countries. Cross-national variation in the gender gap in depression. Social science & medicine. 2010 Jul 1; 71(2): 305–13.
184. van den Bemt L, Schermer T, Bor H, Smink R, van Weel-Baumgarten E, Lucassen P, van Weel C. The risk for depression comorbidity in patients with COPD. Chest. 2009 Jan 1; 135(1): 108–14.
185. Veenhoven R. The four Qualities of life Ordering concepts and measures of the good life. J Happiness Stud. 2000; 1(1): 1–39.
186. Wang K, DiChiacchio T, Fang W, Lander L, Feinberg J, Xie C, Winstanley EL, Piamjariyakul U. Longitudinal study of impact of medication for opioid use disorder on Hamilton Depression Rating Scale. Journal of Affective Disorders. 2022 Jan 15;297:148-55.
187. von Wietersheim J, Kessler H. Psychotherapy with chronic inflammatory bowel disease patients: a review. Inflammatory bowel diseases. 2006 Dec 1; 12(12): 1175–84.
188. Wagena E, Kant I, van Amelsvoort LG, et al. Risk of depression and anxiety in employees with chronic bronchitis: the modifying effect of cigarette smoking. Psychosom Med. 2004; 66: 729–734.
189. Waraich P, Goldner EM, Somers JM, Hsu L. Prevalence and incidence studies of mood disorders: a systematic review of the literature. The Canadian Journal of Psychiatry. 2004 Feb; 49(2): 124–38.
190. WHO. The World Health Organization Quality of Life Assessment –WHO-QoL, 1998.
191. WHO. Chronic obstructive pulmonary disease (COPD). Available at https://www.who.int/news-room/fact-sheets/detail/chronic-obstructive-pulmonary-disease-(copd) Published June 21, 2021. Accessed: July 24, 2021.
192. WHO. Depression and other common mental disorders: global health estimates. World Health Organization. Geneva. 2017. Available at https://apps.who.int/iris/handle/10665/254610
193. WHO. Fact sheet on Sustainable Development Goals (SDGs): health targets. Mental health. 2018.

194. WHO. The global burden of disease: 2004 update. 2004. Available at http://www.who.int/entity/healthinfo/global_burden_disease/GBD_report_2004update_full.pdf.
195. WHO. The ICD-10 classification of mental and behavioural disorders: clinical descriptions and diagnostic guidelines. World Health Organization; 1992.
196. WHO. WHOQOL-BREF: introduction, administration, scoring and generic version of the assessment: field trial version, December 1996: Geneva: World Health Organization; 1996.
197. WHO. World Health Organization. 2021. World health statistics 2021: monitoring health for the SDGs, sustainable development goals. Available at https://www.who.int/publications/i/item/9789240027053
198. WHO. World Health Organization. 2022. World health statistics 2022: monitoring health for the SDGs, sustainable development goals. Available at https://www.who.int/publications/i/item/9789240051157
199. Wijesinghe M, Perrin K, Healy B, Hart K, Clay J, Weatherall M, Beasley R. Pre-hospital oxygen therapy in acute exacerbations of chronic obstructive pulmonary disease. Internal medicine journal. 2011 Aug; 41(8): 618–22.
200. Williams LJ, Pasco JA, Jackson H, Kiropoulos L, Stuart AL, Jacka FN, Berk M. Depression as a risk factor for fracture in women: a 10 year longitudinal study. Journal of affective disorders. 2016 Mar 1; 192: 34–40.
201. Wojewódzka-Wiewiórska A, Kłoczko-Gajewska A, Sulewski P. Between the social and economic dimensions of sustainability in rural areas—in search of farmers' quality of life. Sustainability. 2019 Dec 23; 12(1): 148.
202. Wong TS, Xiang YT, Tsoh J, Ungvari GS, Ko FW, Hui DS, Chiu HF. Depressive disorders in older patients with chronic obstructive pulmonary disease (COPD) in Hong Kong: a controlled study. Aging & mental health. 2014 Jul 4; 18(5): 588–92.
203. Yao HM, Xiao RS, Cao PL, Wang XL, Zuo W, Zhang W. Risk factors for depression in patients with chronic obstructive pulmonary disease. World Journal of Psychiatry. 2020 Apr 4; 10(4): 59.
204. Yin HL, Yin SQ, Lin QY, Xu Y, Xu HW, Liu T. Prevalence of comorbidities in chronic obstructive pulmonary disease patients: a meta-analysis. Medicine. 2017 May; 96(19).
205. Yohannes AM, Alexopoulos GS. Depression and anxiety in patients with COPD. European Respiratory Review. 2014 Sep 1; 23(133): 345–9.
206. Yohannes AM, Hann M, Sibbald B. The management of depressive symptoms in patients with COPD: a postal survey of general practitioners. Primary health care research & development. 2011 Jul; 12(3): 237–44.

207. Yohannes AM, Jin JW, Kunik ME. Benefit–risk assessment of psychotropic drugs in older patients with chronic obstructive pulmonary disease. Drugs & Aging. 2022 May; 39(5): 323–32.
208. Yohannes AM, Leroi I. Pharmacological therapy and anxiolytics in patients with respiratory diseases. Depression and anxiety in patients with chronic respiratory diseases. 2017: 167–82
209. Yoshida T, Tuder RM. Pathobiology of cigarette smoke-induced chronic obstructive pulmonary disease. Physiological reviews. 2007 Jul; 87(3): 1047–82.
210. Zapf W, Glatzer W. German Social Report: Living Conditions and Subjective Well-Being. Soc Indic Res. 1984; 19: 1–171.
211. Zareifopoulos N, Bellou A, Spiropoulou A, Spiropoulos K. Prevalence, contribution to disease burden and management of comorbid depression and anxiety in chronic obstructive pulmonary disease: a narrative review. COPD J Chronic Obstr Pulm Dis. 2019; 16(5–6): 406–417. doi:10.1080/15412555.2019.1679102
212. Zdravković M, Krotin M, Deljanin-Ilić M, Zdravković D. Merenje kvaliteta života bolesnika sa kardiovaskularnim oboljenjima. Medicinski pregled. 2010; 9: 10.
213. Zhou X, Baron RM, Hardin M, et al. Identification of a chronic obstructive pulmonary disease genetic determinant that regulates HHIP. Hum Mol Genet 2012; 21: 1325.
214. Zuo M, Huang Y, Ma W, Xue Z, Zhang J, Gong Y, Che L. Expert recommendations for tracheal intubation in critically ill patients with noval coronavirus disease 2019. Chinese Medical Sciences Journal. 2020 Jun 1; 35(2): 105–9.

Editors

Goran Mihajlović

MD, MSc, PhD, Psychiatrist, Full Professor,

Faculty of Medical Sciences, University of Kragujevac, Serbia

Head, Department of Affective Disorders,

Clinic for Psychiatry, University Clinical Center Kragujevac

Member of the Presidency of the Serbian Medical Association

E-mail: drgoranmih@gmail.com

Ivana Jelić

MD, PhD, Psychiatrist

Primary Health Care Kragujevac, Serbia

Specialist consulting workplace of Psychiatry in Primary Care, Kragujevac, Serbia

Faculty of Medical Sciences, University of Kragujevac, Serbia

E-mail: jelicivana82@yahoo.com

Hamilton Rating Scale for Depression (HDRS)

The HDRS (also known as the HAM-D [Hamilton J et al., 1967]) is the most widely used clinician-administered depression assessment scale. The original version contains 17 items (HDRS17) pertaining to symptoms of depression experienced over the past week (e.g. [Wang K et al., 2022; Akpinar K et al., Shadid A. et al., 2011]). It consists of 17 questions with the possibility of ranking the answers on a four-point scale from 0 to 3, with higher values on the scale indicating the presence of more intense depressive symptoms. The total score is calculated by simply adding all the answers, and the total values range from 0 to 63. The scale is widely used in research and in everyday work with patients suffering from depression. It can also be used with psychiatric, non-psychiatric patients, and healthy populations.

Development of a rating scale for primary depressive illness. Br J Soc Clin Psychol 1967; 6(4): 278–296.

Hamilton Depression Rating Scale (HAM-D)

Name: ______________________ Date: ____________

The HAM-D is designed to rate the severity of depression in patients. Although it contains 21 areas, calculate the patient's score on the first 17 answers.

(To be administered by a health care professional)

☐ **1. DEPRESSED MOOD** (Gloomy attitude, pessimism about the future, feeling of sadness, tendency to weep)

0 = Absent
1 = Sadness, etc.
2 = Occasional weeping
3 = Frequent weeping
4 = Extreme symptoms

☐ **2. FEELINGS OF GUILT**

0 = Absent
1 = Self-reproach, feels he/she has let people down
2 = Ideas of guilt
3 = Present illness is a punishment; delusions of guilt
4 = Hallucinations of guilt

☐ **3. SUICIDE**

0 = Absent
1 = Feels life is not worth living
2 = Wishes he/she were dead
3 = Suicidal ideas or gestures
4 = Attempts at suicide

☐ **4. INSOMNIA - Initial** (Difficulty in falling asleep)

0 = Absent
1 = Occasional
2 = Frequent

☐ **5. INSOMNIA - Middle** ((Complains of being restless and disturbed during the night. Waking during the night.)

0 = Absent
1 = Occasional
2 = Frequent

☐ **6. INSOMNIA - Delayed** (Waking in early hours of the morning and unable to fall asleep again)

0 = Absent
1 = Occasional
2 = Frequent

☐ **7. WORK AND INTERESTS**

0 = No difficulty
1 = Feelings of incapacity, listlessness, indecision and vacillation
2 = Loss of interest in hobbies, decreased social activities
3 = Productivity decreased
4 = Unable to work. Stopped working because of present illness only. (Absence from work after treatment or recovery may rate a lower score).

☐ **8. RETARDATION** (Slowness of thought, speech, and activity; apathy; stupor.)

0 = Absent
1 = Slight retardation at interview
2 = Obvious retardation at interview
3 = Interview difficult
4 = Complete stupor

☐ **9. AGITATION** (Restlessness associated with anxiety.)

0 = Absent
1 = Occasional
2 = Frequent

☐ **10. ANXIETY - PSYCHIC**

0 = No difficulty
1 = Tension and irritability
2 = Worrying about minor matters
3 = Apprehensive attitude
4 = Fears

Hamilton Depression Rating Scale (HAM-D)

☐ **11. ANXIETY - SOMATIC** (Gastrointestinal, indigestion Cardiovascular, palpitation, Headaches Respiratory, Genito-urinary, etc.)

0 = Absent
1 = Mild
2 = Moderate
3 = Severe
4 = Incapacitating

☐ **12. SOMATIC SYMPTOMS - GASTROINTESTINAL** (Loss of appetite , heavy feeling in abdomen; constipation)

0 = Absent
1 = Mild
2 = Severe

☐ **13. SOMATIC SYMPTOMS - GENERAL** (Heaviness in limbs, back or head; diffuse backache; loss of energy and fatiguability)

0 = Absent
1 = Mild
2 = Severe

☐ **14. GENITAL SYMPTOMS** (Loss of libido, menstrual disturbances)

0 = Absent
1 = Mild
2 = Severe

☐ **15. HYPOCHONDRIASIS**

0 = Not present
1 = Self-absorption (bodily)
2 = Preoccupation with health
3 = Querulous attitude
4 = Hypochondriacal delusions

☐ **16. WEIGHT LOSS**

0 = No weight loss
1 = Slight
2 = Obvious or severe

☐ **17. INSIGHT (Insight must be interpreted in terms of patient's understanding and background.)**

0 = No loss
1 = Partial or doubtful loss
2 = Loss of insight

TOTAL ITEMS 1 TO 17: ____________
0 - 7 = Normal
8 - 13 = Mild Depression
14-18 = Moderate Depression 1
9 - 22 = Severe Depression
> 23 = Very Severe Depression

☐ **18. DIURNAL VARIATION** (Symptoms worse in morning or evening. Note which it is.)

0 = No variation
1 = Mild variation; AM (   ) PM (   )
2 = Severe variation; AM (   ) PM (   )

☐ **19. DEPERSONALIZATION AND DEREALIZATION** (feelings of unreality, nihilistic ideas)

0 = Absent
1 = Mild
2 = Moderate
3 = Severe
4 = Incapacitating

☐ **20. PARANOID SYMPTOMS** (Not with a depressive quality)

0 = None
1 = Suspicious 2 = Ideas of reference
3 = Delusions of reference and persecution
4 = Hallucinations, persecutory

☐ **21. OBSESSIONAL SYMPTOMS** (Obsessive thoughts and compulsions against which the patient struggles)

0 = Absent
1 = Mild
2 = Severe

Reference: Hamilton M. A rating scale for depression. J Neurol Neurosurg Psychiatry 1960; 23:56–62

Q-LES-Q-SF – Quality of Life and Life Satisfaction Questionnaire, Short Form

The Q-LES-Q-SF [Endicott J et al., 1993] is a 14-item questionnaire designed to measure satisfaction with physical health, social relationships, ability to function in daily life, physical mobility, mood, family relationships, sexual drive and interest, ability to engage in hobbies, work, leisure and household activities, economic status, living/housing situation, vision, and general well-being. Each of the 14 items is rated on a 1–5-point scale, indicating the degree of enjoyment or satisfaction experienced during the past week. The minimum score is 0 and the maximum score is 100, with higher scores indicating a better quality of life. Higher Q-LES-Q-SF scores indicate greater satisfaction. The instrument also includes two additional items, not included in the total score [Lee YT et al., 2014; Stevanovic D, 2013], that measure satisfaction with medication and overall satisfaction with life. As the French version of the Q-LES-Q-SF has been shown to provide valid and reliable clinical assessments of health status, it was also used in our study. The reliability of the Q-LES-Q-SF, i.e. The reliability of the scales derived from the Q-LES-Q-SF questionnaire feature groups was tested using Cronbach's analysis, which confirmed the internal consistency of the questions and the reliability of the measuring instrument [303–305]. This questionnaire has shown high reliability in our environment, and not only in chronic diseases. There are an increasing number of studies being conducted in clinical centers in Serbia, thus indicating the relevance of this topic in our country [Stevanovic D, 2013, Bourion-Bédès S et al., 2015].

Name:______________________________ Date:______________

Quality of Life Enjoyment and Satisfaction Questionnaire – Short Form (Q-LES-Q-SF)

Taking everything into consideration, during the past week how satisfied have you been with your.........

	Very Poor	Poor	Fair	Good	Very Good
.....physical health?	☐ 1	☐ 2	☐ 3	☐ 4	☐ 5
.....mood?	☐ 1	☐ 2	☐ 3	☐ 4	☐ 5
.....work?	☐ 1	☐ 2	☐ 3	☐ 4	☐ 5
.....household activities?	☐ 1	☐ 2	☐ 3	☐ 4	☐ 5
.....social relationships?	☐ 1	☐ 2	☐ 3	☐ 4	☐ 5
.....family relationships?	☐ 1	☐ 2	☐ 3	☐ 4	☐ 5
.....leisure time activities?	☐ 1	☐ 2	☐ 3	☐ 4	☐ 5
.....ability to function in daily life?	☐ 1	☐ 2	☐ 3	☐ 4	☐ 5
.....sexual drive, interest and/or performance?*	☐ 1	☐ 2	☐ 3	☐ 4	☐ 5
.....economic status?	☐ 1	☐ 2	☐ 3	☐ 4	☐ 5
.....living/housing situation?*	☐ 1	☐ 2	☐ 3	☐ 4	☐ 5
.....ability to get around physically without feeling dizzy or unsteady or falling?*	☐ 1	☐ 2	☐ 3	☐ 4	☐ 5
.....your vision in terms of ability to do work or hobbies?*	☐ 1	☐ 2	☐ 3	☐ 4	☐ 5
.....overall sense of well being?	☐ 1	☐ 2	☐ 3	☐ 4	☐ 5
.....medication? (If not taking any, check here ☐ and leave item blank.)	☐ 1	☐ 2	☐ 3	☐ 4	☐ 5
.....How would you rate your overall life satisfaction and contentment during the past week?	☐ 1	☐ 2	☐ 3	☐ 4	☐ 5

*If satisfaction is very poor, poor or fair on these items, please UNDERLINE the factor(s) associated with a lack of satisfaction.

www.ingramcontent.com/pod-product-compliance
Lightning Source LLC
LaVergne TN
LVHW022312200926
848481LV00004B/1299
9798899660443